Recent Advances in Animal Nutrition

2014

P.C. Garnsworthy, PhD
J. Wiseman, PhD
University of Nottingham

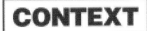

Context Products Ltd
53 Mill Street, Packington
Leicestershire, LE65 1WN, United Kingdom
www.contextbookshop.com

First published 2015

British Library Cataloguing in Publication Data
Recent Advances in Animal Nutrition - 2014

ISBN 9781899043699
ISSN 0269-5642

Disclaimer

Preface

The 46th University of Nottingham Feed Conference was held at the School of Biosciences, Sutton Bonington Campus, 24th – 25th June 2014. The Conference was divided into sessions that covered areas of topical interest to the animal feed industry. These sessions were Ruminants, General Issues, and Non-ruminants.

The Ruminant section is concerned with improving efficiency of dairy systems. The first chapter discusses effects of nutrition on metabolic health and reproduction. The second highlights the role of carnitine in energy metabolism. The third and fourth chapters provide updates on responses to dietary starch and amino acids. The fifth reviews techniques for manipulating rumen fermentation. The sixth chapter explains how to optimise calf and heifer rearing to enhance lifetime performance.

The General section starts with a chapter on recent developments in feed technology across species. The second explores the potential use of insects for animal feed. The third discusses important indicators of animal health and welfare.

The non-ruminant section is concerned with health and nutrition of pigs and poultry. The first chapter describes the impact of porcine reproductive and respiratory syndrome virus. The second provides guidance on how to improve performance at the lower end of the production scale. The third reviews use of fermented feeds for pigs. The fourth discusses updates from the 2012 NRC guidelines. The fifth shows how processing affects feed efficiency in pigs and poultry. The final chapter provides an overview of current thinking on gilt management and nutrition.

We would like to thank all speakers for their presentations and written papers, which have maintained the high standards and international standing of the Nottingham Feed Conference. We are grateful to all those members of the feed industry who provided suggestions and assistance in developing the conference programme. We would also like to acknowledge the input of those who helped us to chair sessions (Mike Wilkinson and Tim Parr) and the administrative (managed by Sheila Northover and Kathy Lawson), catering and support staff who ensure the smooth running of the conference. We would like to thank our sponsors (listed on next page). Finally we would like to thank the delegates who made valuable contributions both to the discussion sessions and the general atmosphere of the meeting.

P.C. Garnsworthy
J. Wiseman

Sponsors

The 2014 Nottingham Feed Conference was kindly sponsored by:

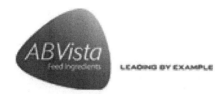

AB Vista Feed Ingredients (http://www.abvista.com/)

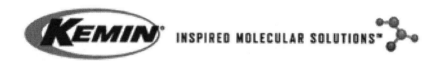

Kemin (http://www.kemin.com/)

CONTENTS

1

Managing Nutrition to Improve the Metabolic Health and Reproduction of Dairy Cows

JOS NOORDHUIZEN

DVM, PhD, former Diplomate of the ECVPH and the ECBHM. School of Agriculture and Veterinary Science, Charles Sturt University, Wagga Wagga, NSW, Australia; VACQA-international consultancies, France

Introduction

Transition cow management is currently considered as the key factor for subsequent adequate milk productivity, dairy cow health and reproduction. Transition cow management is a container term. It comprises different aspects of farm management, even including the nutrition at the end of lactation and during the dry period, as well as the cows' health status during the latter periods, but most of all it comprises the nutrition during about the last 20 days antepartum and the first 30 days postpartum, the health status of the cows during these weeks, and husbandry factors such as housing and barn climate, as well as cow comfort elements. Transition cow management should prepare the cow in such a way that she would be able to adequately counteract the different periods of high risk between calving and day 100 postpartum. In this context, risks refer to metabolic, other health and reproductive disorders during the transition period. Inadequate transition management leads to a whole spectrum of subclinical and clinical health, reproduction and milk production disorders.

This paper addresses issues of transition cow management and the respective risk periods after calving. These risk periods comprise health and fertility disorders. Ultimately, management measures to better control and possibly prevent disorders in the period between calving and day 100 postpartum are discussed.

Transition cow management

The transition period is schematically described in Figure 1. This Figure illustrates the different physiological and pathophysiological processes, major events in this period, and the respective relevant hazards. The transition period comprises 20 days close-up, the calving event, and the first 30 days in milk. The ultimate objective of transition cow management is to adequately prepare the cow for optimal feed intake and metabolism, health, production and reproduction prior to, around and after calving. Basically, when speaking about the "cow" in this context, we should rather speak about the "rumen" (microflora, rumen layers, papillae, motility, pH, fatty acid ratio). Transition cow management is about adaptation processes in the cow, which – along with rumen issues – are influenced by external factors such stressors, husbandry and cow comfort (Kumar-Dubey, 2012; Cardoso *et al.*, 2013).

The following physiological and patho-physiological processes take place around parturition (Figure1, Label 1). After a decrease in feed intake in the last week antepartum, the neuro-endocrinological preparation for parturition, the start of colostrum production, and parturition itself, the cow enters a state of relative lack of energy (uptake is less than demand). Lack of energy is aggravated by the increasing milk yield after parturition. The cow is in a negative energy balance (NEB), which sometimes is severe and/or of long duration. In most cases the interval from parturition to resumption of positive energy balance is, on average, 45 days; adult cows and heifers showing no difference (SD 21 days; Grummer, 2006).

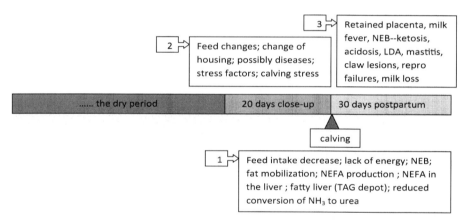

Figure 1. The transition period, with different processes (1), possible events (2) and potential subsequent hazards (3) (adapted after Kumar-Dubey, 2012). NEB= negative energy balance; LDA= left abomasal displacement; NEFA= non-esterified fatty acids; TAG= triacylglycerides

In order to adapt to NEB, the cow mobilises energy from adipose tissues through lipolysis. Non-esterified fatty acids (NEFA) and triacylglycerides (TAG) are produced also, the latter rapidly infiltrating the liver during and after parturition (Vanden Top *et al.*, 1995). Studies using liver biopsies have shown that up to 50% of cows experience fatty liver before parturition; other studies point to a variation of 15 to 35% (Rehage *et al.*, 2012). Fatty liver leads to "type II ketosis" at around 5 to 15 days postpartum. A "type I ketosis" (without fatty liver) occurs at 3 to 6 weeks postpartum (Oetzel, 2004 in LeBlanc, 2012). The clinical form of ketosis is acetonaemia, which has a reported prevalence of around 1%. The liver plays a key role in the adaptation process, but other adaptation factors contribute as well (e.g. leptin, resistin, gut peptides, Gh-relin, oesteocalcin; Bradford, 2011). Through beta-oxidation, acetyl-co-enzyme A and the Krebs cycle, finally aceto-acetate is produced. The end-point is production of ketone bodies leading to ketosis and possibly acetonaemia. Acetonaemia can be worsened by several events (Figure1, Label 2): an over-condition in the dry period (Body condition score (BCS) > 3.5), a fatty liver, a persistent decrease in feed intake, a ketogenic ration, diseases and various stressors in the transition period or around parturition. These events may trigger subsequent hazards for health, productivity and reproduction (Figure1, Label 3). Energy balance recovery is influenced much more by energy concentration of the ration than by milk production level (Grummer, 2006). Due to a hampered liver function (fatty liver increases the risk of liver failure fivefold, at least partly due to peroxidative processes), protein metabolism may be affected also, which is shown by poor conversion of ammonia to urea. Cows with fatty liver and loss of liver function show a dramatic insulin resistance (Rehage *et al.*, 2012). Inflammatory diseases postpartum, such as metritis, provoke release of cytokines. These cytokines depress insulin secretion and responsiveness; both have a negative effect on subsequent metabolism and reproduction (Kerestes *et al.*, 2009, in Cardoso *et al.*, 2013). When ruminal acidosis occurs in the same period postpartum, various consequences may be detected. During subacute ruminal acidosis (SARA) bacterial immunogens such as lipopolysaccharides (LPS) are released in the rumen and intestines (Dong *et al.*, 2001). These LPS are translocated to the blood and provoke an immune response (increase of neutrophils, serum amyloid A, haptoglobins, LPS binding protein, C-reactive protein). The LPS affect metabolism by increasing blood glucose, NEFA, and reactive oxygen species (cytotoxic for e.g. mammary gland cells) while feed intake decreases. Low ruminal pH was associated with dystocia, metritis and lameness postpartum. A low ruminal pH was found in cows with a low serum-BHB level and a high BCS loss postpartum; conception rate was decreased as well (Inchaisri *et al.*, 2014). One explanation is that ruminal acidosis may lead to metabolic acidosis which leads to further outcomes (oxidative stress; inflammatory response; increased blood cortisol; hampered liver function; loss of uterine contractility; decrease in insulin secretion).

An important marker for transition cow management is the degree of feed intake reduction. Commonly feed intake is reduced to a certain extent during the last days or week before calving and immediately after calving (Grummer, 2006; DeKruif *et al.*, 1998; Zom, personal communication, 2014).

Transition management parameters in the field

Feed intake decrease is influenced by several factors, the most important of which are listed in Table 1 (Interact AgriManagement, 2004 in Noordhuizen, 2012).

The different domains and factors, as listed in Table 1, point to the complexity of transition cow management which is possibly the explanation for the phenomenon that some farmers are very successful in this management while others are not. Several of these domains and factors have 'read out' parameters in the field. Body condition score is one example; at end of lactation 3.0 to 3.5, in the dry period 3.5 to 3.0. Others are rumen fill score (RF), faeces consistency score (FC), undigested fibres in faeces (UF) (Zaaijer & Noordhuizen, 2003). Feed bunk space should be 75 cm per cow; for high yielding cows even 90 cm. Total width of available drinking place in the barn or pasture should be 450 cm for 100 cows, and may be double in warm summer seasons, and troughs must be well positioned throughout the barn and in pasture. Rumination frequency in the herd should be > 75% of the cows (if not eating). The diurnal feeding pattern in cows is influenced mostly by time of feeding, and less by feed push-ups or milking (DeVries, 2011). Giving smaller but

Table 1. Overview of domains and factors per domain which may impact on the extent of feed intake reduction before and after parturition (adapted after Interact AgriManagement, 2004, in Noordhuizen, 2012)

Domain	Factors
Dry period management	Manner of preparation of cows (BCS 3.0-3.5 max)
	Presence/absence of far-off and close-up cow groups
	Cow comfort conditions (see below)
Feeding	Palatability of grass/maize (silage)
	Fibre content in grass/maize (silage)
	Other feed (by)products
Feeding management	Feeding according to standards
	Freshness and quality of rations fed
	Rations based on forage analysis
	Total Mixed Ration (TMR) mixing and mixing time
	Supply of feed over the day
	Speed of increase in concentrates supply after parturition
	Feed bunk space per cow and heifer
	Animal density (< or > 100%) and presence of cow groups
Claw and leg health	Presence of infectious & non-infectious claw lesions
	Presence of hock lesions
Cow comfort	Barn ventilation conditions
	Barn light regimen applied
	Conditions and surface of exercise area behind feed rack
	Cubicle design and maintenance, including bedding
	Competition for cubicles, feeding places, escape
	Drinking water troughs (barn/pasture) number, position
	Water quality (chemical; micro-biological)
	Water cleanness
	Water distribution system (adults one; youngstock one)

more frequent meals is beneficial for feed intake, mobility and health. Selection by cows of grains or concentrates from TMR rations can be observed; this will result in a higher risk of SARA and poorer quality of remaining feed for other cows, so should be avoided (Kleen *et al.*, 2003). The increase in concentrates supply after calving should be conducted gradually over a 2 to 3 week period. Water quality should be tested, both in the field (Van Eenige *et al.*, 2013) and in the laboratory, to facilitate supply of water of highest chemical and microbiological quality.

Particular characteristics of inadequate transition cow management are: over-condition (BCS > 3.5) at parturition and fatty liver; decrease of feed intake before and after parturition; occurrence of NEB and ketosis; more or less severe loss of BCS after parturition; various health disorders (ruminal acidosis; milk fever; LDA; mastitis; claw lesions) and reproductive disorders (Bradford, 2011; Butler, 2012; Noordhuizen, 2012).

Effects of adaptation processes and events on metabolic health of cows

Ketosis is a common feature in high yielding dairy cows, partly physiological in nature because of normal adaptation, and partly a pathological process mainly started in the liver (e.g. fatty liver; NEB consequences) or in case of persistent hunger. Ketosis leads to immune depression, which in turn increases the risk of mastitis and infectious claw lesions (Suryasathaporn *et al.*, 2000) and may further contribute to occurrence of LDA and rumen acidosis. Milk yield parameters are affected too: next to a decrease in milk yield, most often increased milk fat and decreased milk protein content can be observed in ketotic cows, while in acidotic cows milk protein content is increased and milk fat content decreased (Noordhuizen, 2012).

Epidemiological studies (LeBlanc, 2012a, 2012b) have shown the relationship between transition cow management parameters and the risk of health disorders after parturition. For example, high serum NEFA concentration around 10 days antepartum, a positive urine test for ketone bodies, high serum betahydroxybuturate (BHB) and low serum calcium levels were each associated with an increased risk of LDA occurrence (Odds Ratio 3.5; 11.8; 2.6; 2.0 respectively), while high serum NEFA and serum cholesterol concentrations were associated with increased risk of retained placenta (Odds Ratio 1.8 and 1.9 respectively). Serum or milk BHB is commonly used as a parameter to diagnose ketosis in groups of cows (herds between 50 and 1000 cows), with an alarm prevalence threshold value of 10% of tested cows and a cut-off value of the test at 100 µmol/l. A sample of 12 to 15 fresh (to detect a ketosis problem) or close-up (to prevent ketosis as much as possible) cows is considered convenient (Dohoo *et al.*, 2003 and Oetzel, 2004, in LeBlanc, 2012a).

Effects of adaptation processes and events on reproductive performance of cows

Although conception rate for adult cows in the USA declined from 66% in 1950 to 51% in 1986 (Smith, 1986 in Grummer, 2006), no change was observed in conception rate for heifers over the same period. The suggestion was that genetics apparently were not responsible for this decline and that other factors were involved. Studies have highlighted energy balance, and as a proxy parameter BCS, as being positively related to services per conception and conception rates (Butler & Smith, 1989; Britt, 1992). Energy status in the transition period is associated with reproductive performance 2 to 4 months later (LeBlanc, 2012a, 2012b). About 60% of cows are anovulatory at 60 days postpartum. Cows that were ketotic in the first week of lactation, were 50% more likely to be in anoestrus around 60 days postpartum (Walsh, 2006, in LeBlanc, 2012a). Ketosis is associated with a 50% reduction in probability of pregnancy at first insemination. Oocytes harvested between 80 and 140 days postpartum in an *in vitro* study (Wensing *et al.*, 1997, in Cardoso *et al.*, 2013) showed a lowered development stage in cows with an induced hepatic lipidosis postpartum. Epidemiological evidence showed that among cows there is individual variation with respect to liver oxidative, storage and export capacity (Jorritsma *et al.*, 2003, in Cardoso *et al.*, 2013). This phenomenon may, at least partly, explain differences in reproductive performance.

Fresh cows losing more than one unit BCS had longer intervals from parturition to first ovulation, to first observed heat, and to first AI, and lower conception rate, than cows with less BCS loss. Milk production did not differ significantly between these groups, nor did plasma progesterone concentration during the first two oestrous cycles, but plasma progesterone concentration differed significantly during the third, fourth and fifth cycles. This finding supports the idea that follicle development is, at least partly, dependent on energy status of the cow. Butler (2012) reported a strong association between early postpartum resumption of ovulatory cycles and pregnancy rate. Another study pointed to the strong positive relationship (R^2 0.72) between days to NEB nadir and days to first ovulation (Butler & Canfield, 1989; Grummer, 2006). Delay in first ovulation is associated with decreased conception rate and increased interval from parturition to conception.

Preventive and control measures

Some basic management measures have been highlighted above. Other preventive and control measures can be derived from the issues listed in Table 1. Cow comfort plays, next to nutrition, a paramount role. Cow comfort comprises the best possible environment for cows during the transition period and thereafter. It includes:

optimal housing and barn climate; optimal feed and feeding management, as well as drinking water availability and quality; optimal health status (mainly claw health); and species-specific behaviour expression opportunities such as grooming (Noordhuizen & Lievaart, 2005).

Given the difference in occurrence between type I and type II ketosis, their prevention and control are slightly different. When ketosis monitoring points to a problem in the first two weeks of lactation, prevention should focus on managing BCS in the close-up period at a level of 3.0 to 3.5 (hence to avoid all over-conditioning); furthermore, feed intake around parturition should be enhanced. Prevention for type II ketosis should focus primarily on stabilising a good feed intake, both before and after parturition. The classic treatment measures, such as propylene glycol and dexamethasone, should be considered for affected cows. Moreover, dexamethasone has been reported to decrease plasma ammonia levels and to increase plasma lysine and tyrosine (Rehage *et al.*, 2012). Supplementation with vitamin E, selenium or other antioxidative products could be indicated if liver failure (peroxidative processes) is suspected. The influence of dietary fat (quantity; quality; source) in the postpartum ration appears to be a continuous issue for debate (Grummer, 2006; Garnsworthy, 2012).

Choline supplementation is another current topic. Choline (*trimethyl ethanol amine*) is present in rumen bacteria and protozoa; the highest flow is in the duodenum. Choline is a key factor for the synthesis of phospatidyl-choline and acetylcholine (neurotransmitter). Phospatidyl-choline is relevant for lipid absorption, cell membrane structure, lipoprotein synthesis, and is essential for VLDL formation which contributes to transportation of TAG from the liver. Rations rich in concentrates may trigger ruminal acidosis, by which protozoa decrease and, hence, also the choline level. Cows with high milk yield are basically in a constant deficiency of the essential choline (Santos & Lima, 2009). Choline is known to influence carnitine synthesis positively, which mediates fat metabolism; ample intervention field study results on choline with a proven positive effect are not yet available (Kumar-Dubey, 2012). Various experimental studies point to a fatty liver preventive effect and a reduction of fat mobilization and ketosis (from 28.8% to 10.7%); close-up period supplementation of rumen-protected choline increased feed intake postpartum (Lima *et al.*, 2007 in Santos & Lima, 2009).

With regard to the ration during the transition period, various studies with variable outcomes have been published. Interesting studies refer to the energy density of the ration (Rabelo & Rezende, 2005; Rastani *et al.* in Grummer, 2006). In these studies, low-energy rations (1.50 Mcal NE/kg) during the first 4 weeks of the dry period were followed by moderate-energy (1.69 Mcal NE/kg) rations during the last 4 weeks dry, and high energy rations (1.75 Mcal NE/kg) after parturition. Cows in this study hardly showed a negative energy balance antepartum. Low energy with high fibre in the ration did not affect duration or extent of NEB. Restricted feeding in the dry period, and, next during the far-off period, in particular in the close-up period, has been addressed by Cardoso *et al.* (2013). Cows on restricted energy diets (less than or equal to recommendation) in the close-up period became pregnant 10 days earlier than cows fed high energy diets (energy density based on net energy for lactation, NE_L); the former cows had eaten more and better after parturition than the latter cows. Moreover, BCS loss after parturition was less for cows fed restricted energy diets as compared to cows fed high energy diets; NEFA concentrations postpartum were lower and glucose levels higher in restricted energy fed cows than in high energy fed cows. Preliminary results of an extensive field study in the Netherlands point to the fact that feed intake capacity of close-up cows has been overestimated (10%) in the past decades; moreover, around parturition another drop of feed intake capacity (15%) was determined (Zom *et al.*, 2014). These findings are in agreement with the philosophy of restricted or controlled energy feeding mentioned above. Since it is known that concentrations of amino acids such as lysine, isoleucine and tyrosine are decreased in ketotic cows, supplementation of these could be considered. Excessive protein contents in the ration should be avoided in order to reduce ammonia overload to the (possibly damaged) liver. Oocyte quality postpartum may be improved by a ration low in carbohydrates and/or high in fat, but on the other hand, such a ration could hamper the restart of oestrous cycles (Garnsworthy, 2012). These issues concerning ration energy and fat content make the discussion complex and introduce new decisions to be made when designing ration composition. Possibly, the feed industry could think about different diets for specific stages of lactation, as is already the case in pig husbandry.

The transition period also shows a change in calcium demand for the colostrum and milk production to come. When calcium supply does not meet demand, disorders such as milk fever may occur (incidence 5%; prevalence in first lactation heifers 25%, in adult cows 41% to 54% in the USA; Silva del Rio, 2014). Calcium is relevant for both muscle contractility and immune function. Calcium deficiency has been associated with retained placenta, metritis, subfertility, mastitis, decreased rumen and abomasum motility, and abomasal displacement. Some dairy farms could consider investigating the dietary cation-anion difference (DCAD) in the herd. DCAD reflects the cow's status in sodium, potassium, chlorides and sulphate; the first two components are cationic, the last two are anionic. A negative DCAD in dry cows is beneficial for the prevention of parathyroid hormone receptor function loss; this parathyroid hormone is a key in calcium metabolism. Farmers could consider supplementation of anionic salts to close-up cows. Anionic salts comprise chlorides, sulphates and or phosphates; they are expensive and unpalatable and a potential threat to the environment; their use should be limited. But these anionic compounds can also be found in certain feedstuffs: brewer's grains; cereals; rapeseed; beet pulp. A ration rich in grass- and maize (silage) for close-up cows is far too positive in DCAD.

A close-up cow DCAD can be evaluated by testing the cows' urine pH: in Holstein cows urine pH values should be between 6.2 and 6.8, in Jersey cows between 5.8 and 6.3. Lactating cows need a positive DCAD, hence relatively more sodium and potassium. These components can be found in grass and maize (silage), sugar beets; hay and lucerne (Silva del Rio, 2014).

Concluding remarks

Negative energy balance and ketosis are two example parameters of a failed transition management. Their situation may be aggravated by other factors, such as over-condition, fatty liver, poor cow comfort and diseases around parturition like ruminal acidosis. The consequences are manifold, both in health disorders, milk production losses and poor reproductive performance, resulting in large economic losses on the farm. Therefore, all possible preventive and control measures should be considered.

With respect to the ration in the dry period and after parturition, the issue of controlled or restricted energy content in the far-off period, as well as in the close-up period deserves further attention to better overcome the situation of NEB and ketosis, as well as their consequences in health and reproduction (Rabelo & Rezende, 2005; Cardoso *et al.*, 2013). The same is valid for the postulate of Garnsworthy (2012) regarding a ration low in carbohydrates and/or high in fat to improve oocyte quality; which unfortunately limits the restart of oestrous cyclicity. The feed industry should prioritize these issues in their research for best possible ration formulation for specific lactation stages. Other issues which may be considered when dealing with failing transition performance regards the calcium status of dry and fresh cows, the dietary cation-anion difference, and the supplementation of choline (Santos & Lima, 2009).

References

Bradford, B.J. (2011). The endocrine network: a growing list of hormones regulating transition cow metabolism. In: *Proc. of the Canadian Nutrition Conference*. pp 37-43

Britt, J.H. (1992). Reproductive efficiency in dairy cattle as related to nutrition and environment. In: *Proc. of the Advanced Nutrition seminar for feed professionals*. University of Wisconsin, USA, pp 30

Butler, W.R., Canfield, R.W. (1989). Interrelationships between energy balance and postpartum reproduction. In: *Proc. of the Cornell Nutrition Conference for Feed Manufacturers*, Cornell University, USA

Butler, W.R., (2000). Nutritional interactions with reproductive performance in dairy cattle. *Animal Reproduction Science* **60/61**: 449-457

Butler, W.R. (2012). The role of energy balance and metabolism on reproduction of dairy cows.

In: *Proc. of the 23d Annual Florida Ruminant Nutrition Symposium*, Gainesville, Fl, USA; 31 January and 1 February 2012

Cardoso, F.C., LeBlanc, S.J., Murphy, M.R., Drackley, J.K. (2013.) Prepartum nutritional strategy affects reproductive performance in dairy cows. *Journal of Dairy Science* **96 (9)**: 5859-5871

DeKruif, A., Mansfeld, R., Hoedemakers, M. (1998). *Veterinary herd health programmes for dairy cows*. Enke Ferdinand Verlag, Stuttgart, Germany (in German).

DeVries, T.J. (2011). Not just what dairy cattle are given to eat, but how they eat it. In: *Proc. of the Canadian Nutrition Conference*; pp 73-82

Dong, G., Liu, S., Wu, Y., Lei, C., Zhou, J., Zhang, S. (2011). Diet induced bacterial immunogens in the gastrointestinal tract of dairy cows: impacts on immunity and metabolism. *Acta Vet. Scand.* **53**: 48

Garnsworthy, P.C. (2012). Feeding dairy cows for fertility. In: *Proc. of the Round Table 4 "Balanced nutrition as a prerequisite for optimal cattle health, reproduction and production"* (Editor J. Noordhuizen) during the World Buiatrics Congress, June 2012, Lisbon, Portugal

Grummer, R.R. (2006). Optimization of transition period energy status for improved health and reproduction. In: *Proc. World Buiatrics Congress* 2006 Nice, France (H.Navetat, editor), pp 460-471

Inchaisri, C., Champongsang, S., Noordhuizen, J.P.T.M., Hogeveen, H. (2014). A cow-level association of ruminal pH on body condition score, serum BHB and postpartum disorders in Thai dairy cattle. *Animal Science Journal* (in press, Japan Society of Animal Science).

Interact AgriManagement. (2004). Report on feed and feeding management in Dutch dairy herds (in Dutch), referred to in Noordhuizen (2012) *Dairy Herd Health and Management*, Context Products Ltd, UK.

Jorritsma, R., Wensing, T., Kruip, T.A., Vos, P.L., Noordhuizen J.P. (2003). Metabolic changes in early lactation and impaired reproductive performance in dairy cows. *Veterinary Research* **34**: 11-26

Kleen, J.L., Hooijer, G.A., Rehage, J., Noordhuizen, J.P.T.M. (2003). Subacute ruminal acidosis (SARA) in Dutch dairy herds. *The Veterinary Record* **164**: 681-684

LeBlanc, S.J. (2012a). Optimization of transition period energy status for improved health and reproduction. In: *Proc. World Buiatrics Congress*, Lisbon, Portugal. pp 191-202

LeBlance, S.J. (2012b). Reproductive performance in dairy cattle. In: *Proc. of the Round Table 1 "Reproductive performance in dairy cattle"* (editor J.Noordhuizen) during the World Buiatrics Congress, June 2012, Lisbon, Portugal

Noordhuizen, J.P.T.M., Lievaart, J. (2005).Cow comfort and Cattle welfare. In: *Proc. of the 1ˢᵗ Buiatrissima Congress* (S. Eicher, editor), Bern, Switzerland; 6-11.

Noordhuizen, J.P.T.M. (2012). *Dairy Herd Health and Management*. Context Products Ltd, Packington, UK. 465 pp

Rabelo, E., Rezende, R.L. (2005). Effects of pre- and postfresh transition diets varying in dietary energy density on metabolic status of periparturient dairy cows. *Journal of Dairy Science* **88**: 4375-4383

Rehage, J., Starke, A., Holterschinken, M., Kaske, M. (2012). Hepatic lipidosis: diagnostic tools and individual and herd risk factors. In: *Proc. of the World Buiatrics Congress* (J.Cannas da Silva editor), June 2012, Lisbon, Portugal; pp 69-74

Santos, J.E.P., Lima, F.S. (2009). Feeding rumen-protected choline to transition dairy cows. Publ. of the College of Veterinary Medicine, University of Florida, 149-159. At www.dairy.ifas. ufl.edu consulted 28 February 2014

Silva del Rio, N. (2014). Preventing milk fever with anionic salts. At www.dairyherd.com consulted 18 February 2014.

Suryasathaporn, W., Heuer, C., Stassen, E.N., Schukken, Y.H. (2000). Hyperketonemia and the impairment of udder defense: a review. *Veterinary Research* **31 (4)** 397-412

Van den Top, A.M., Wensing, T., Geelen, M.T.H., Wentink, H. (1995). Time trends of plasma lipids and enzymes synthesizing hepatic triacylglycerol during postpartum development of fatty liver in dairy cows. *Journal of Dairy Science* **78 (10)** 2208-2220.

Van Eenige, E., Counotte, G., Noordhuizen, J.P.T.M. (2013). Drinking water for dairy cattle: always a benefit or a microbiological risk? *Tijdschrijft voor Diergeneeskunde* **138 (2)** 86-97 (with a summary in Dutch)

Zaaijer, D., Noordhuizen, J.P.T.M. (2003). A novel scoring system for monitoring the relationship between nutritional efficiency and fertility in dairy cows. *Irish Veterinary Journal* **56 (3)** 145-151

Zom, R. (2014) Wageningen UR Livestock Research ; Wageningen, The Netherlands ; personal communication

2

Physiological Role of Carnitine in Energy Metabolism, Possible Interplay With Inflammation and Potential Benefits for Dairy Cows

FRANK MENN

Lohmann Animal Health GmbH, Heinz-Lohmann-Straße 4, 27472 Cuxhaven, Germany

Introduction

Carnitine is a naturally occurring substance. It was detected in 1905 as an ingredient in muscle. In contrast to the D-isomer, the L-form plays an essential and crucial role in energy metabolism of human and animal organisms. The function of shuttling long chain fatty acids into the mitochondria for β-oxidation and finally driving the citric acid cycle is well known and published in literature. However, the crucial role of carnitine in regulating carbohydrate and fatty acid metabolism by modulating the acetyl-CoA/CoA ratio in the mitochondria and the consequences for energy metabolism, as well as the link to inflammation, is rarely considered. Carnitine is defined by many scientists as conditionally essential. The aim of this chapter is to elucidate the physiological role of carnitine, the possible interplay with inflammation, and potential benefits for dairy cows.

Endogenous biosynthesis

The chemical structure of L-carnitine is similar to that of amino acids. Endogenous biosynthesis is performed in the liver and kidney. The first metabolite is trimethyllysine (TML). Although lysine and methionine deliver the backbone of this source, the nutritional supply of these amino acids has no impact on the biosynthesis of carnitine. The precursor TML must be provided from body protein following degradation within the scope of protein turnover. Endogenous biosynthesis starts with release of TML from lysosomal protein breakdown (Vaz and Wanders, 2002). Certain physiological conditions (Table 1) may lead to insufficient biosynthesis of carnitine especially under anabolic conditions due to reduced protein degradation. This in turn leads to a lack of TML (Eder, 2013). As metabolism in pregnancy is anabolic it can be assumed that under these conditions endogenous carnitine biosynthesis is reduced due to low availability of precursors, thus generating low plasma carnitine concentrations (Ringseis, 2010). Extensive research in sows proved the benefits of a carnitine supplementation during pregnancy (Eder, 2009).

Table 1: Conditions probably leading to an insufficient endogenous carnitine synthesis (Eder 2013)

Condition	Cause of impaired carnitine synthesis
Pregnancy	Anabolic condition: reduced release of TML from muscle
Obesity	Metabolic syndrome / chronic inflammation?
High fat diet	Increased levels of free fatty acids / chronic inflammation?
Inflammation?	Reduced carnitine synthesis / function?

Functions and mode of action of L-carnitine

The most important functions of L-carnitine in endogenous metabolism are as follows:

- convey medium- and long-chain fatty acids into the mitochondria (shuttle)
- modulate the acetyl-CoA/CoA ratio and thereby regulate carbohydrate- and fatty acid metabolism (buffer)

The mode of action of L-carnitine is based on the following chemical reaction:

$$\text{Acyl-CoA} + \text{Carnitine} \leftrightarrow \text{Acylcarnitine} + \text{CoA}$$

This process can occur in both directions in and outside the mitochondrial matrix depending on requirements (Figure 1). The length of the fatty acid residues is not relevant. Carnitine can thus react with short, medium and long chain fatty acids (Harmeyer and Schlumborn, 1997).

Shuttle function

Fatty acids must be transported into the mitochondrial matrix for β-oxidation to serve as a fuel for energy metabolism. In a first step the fatty acids must be activated by the cofactor CoA. As the inner mitochondrial matrix is impermeable for these activated fatty acids the cofactor CoA must be substituted by carnitine. Acetyl-carnitine can then permeate the mitochondrial matrix. Once inside the mitochondrial matrix, carnitine is in turn replaced by CoA. Medium- and long-chain acyl-CoA is now available for β-oxidation to be broken down to activated acetic acid, acetyl-CoA. Free carnitine leaves the matrix in return with acyl-carnitine for another round (Harmeyer and Schlumborn, 1997; Luppa, 2004).

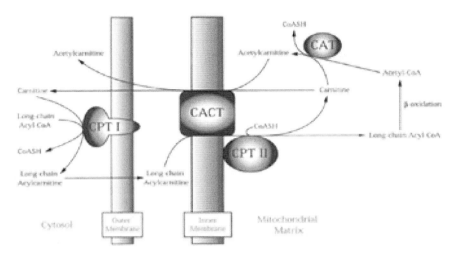

Figure 1. Function of carnitine in transport of mitochondrial long chain fatty acid oxidation and regulation of the mitochondrial acetyl-CoA/CoA ratio (Vaz and Wanders, 2002).

Modulation of Acetyl-CoA/CoA ratio

A shuttle can work repeatedly without being wasted. Hence, the shuttle function of carnitine cannot explain the need for carnitine supplementation. Nevertheless, research in humans and animals has shown that with increasing performance or energy deprivation, the excretion of acetyl-carnitine via urine and milk is increased. In humans renal excretion of carnitine esters increases when fasting or performing endurance sports. These results can be explained by the buffer function, i.e. the modulation of the acetyl-CoA/CoA ratio (Luppa, 2004).

Activated acetic acid at the end of the β-oxidation condenses with oxaloacetate to form citric acid and to fuel the citric acid cycle. Under certain metabolic conditions and diseases, e.g. malnutrition, fasting, diabetes mellitus (Flanagan, Simmons, Vehige, Willcox and Garret, 2010) this metabolic pathway can be overstrained due to excess of fatty acids stemming from the diet or mobilized body fat, leading to a surplus of acetyl-CoA. Most of the CoA in the mitochondria is fixed then to the activated fatty acids and thus not available for other metabolic functions. The enzyme pyruvate dehydrogenase (PDH) in particular plays a crucial role here. This enzyme catalyzes the reaction of pyruvate and its precursors, glucose and glucoplastic substances, with fatty acids. The activity of the PDH depends on free CoA (Luppa, 2004).

If sufficient free carnitine is available in the mitochondrial matrix, carnitine again replaces the CoA in the surplus acetyl-CoA. CoA is released and acetyl-carnitine removed from the mitochondrial matrix in return with free carnitine from the blood. If the capacity of this converse metabolism is exceeded, acetyl-carnitine is excreted via urine and milk. The simultaneously increasing pool of free CoA in the mitochondrial matrix is essential to activate the PDH (Luppa, 2004).

By this mechanism, carnitine strongly reduces intramitochondrial acetyl-CoA levels resulting in a 10- to 20-fold decrease of the acetyl-CoA/CoA ratio (Ringseis, Keller and Eder, 2012).

Effects of carnitine in the Randle cycle

The main fuels for energy metabolism in the organism are glucose and fatty acids reaching the mitochondria via separate pathways. In 1963 Randle, Garland, Hales and Newsholme for the first time described the competition between these two pathways. Increasing glucose oxidation occurs at the cost of fatty acids and vice versa. The mechanism of inhibition of glucose utilization by fatty acid oxidation is explained in Figure 2.

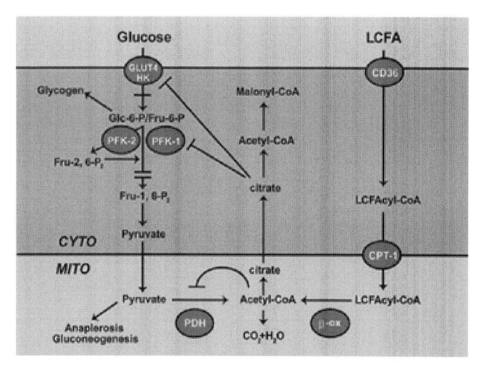

Figure 2. Mechanism of inhibition of glucose utilization by fatty acid oxidation. The extent of inhibition is graded and most severe at the level of PDH. PDH inhibition is caused by acetyl-CoA and NADH accumulation resulting from fatty acid oxidation (Hue and Taegtmeyer, 2009).

This "glucose-fatty acid cycle" or "Randle cycle" does not describe a metabolic cycle like the citric acid cycle, but dynamic interaction between substrates. Competition between the substrates glucose and fatty acids explains why excessive fatty acid oxidation inhibits use of glucose or glucoplastic substances and thereby reduces insulin sensitivity (Wüsten, 1999; Hue and Taegtmeyer, 2009). The buffer function of carnitine, as described above, already implies that carnitine – if available in the mitochondria – can influence this competition of substrates in favour of glucose, as demonstrated in Figure 3. These molecular effects of carnitine in the Randle cycle can thus be compared to an inhibition of the shuttle by antidiabetic drugs like Oxfenicine and Etomoxir, i.e. blocking the entrance to open the gate (Schrauwen, Timmers and Hesselink, 2013).

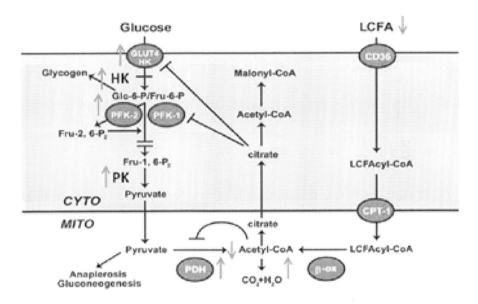

Figure 3. Molecular effects of carnitine in the Randle cycle (Hue and Taegtmeyer, 2009, adapted by Eder 2013).

Regulation of glucose homeostasis and insulin sensitivity

Carnitine supplementation studies in both humans and animals demonstrate an improvement in glucose tolerance, in particular during insulin resistant states (Ringseis *et al.*, 2012). In this review article the authors included 16 human and 9 animal studies with the result that 11 out of these 16 human studies and all animal studies revealed the positive impact of a carnitine supplementation on glucose tolerance. The parameters of glucose tolerance, like fasting plasma glucose, fasting plasma insulin, area under the curve for glucose (AUC_{GLC}), area under the curve for insulin (AUC_{INS}), glucose oxidation rate (GOX) and/or homeostasis model assessment of insulin resistance (HOMA-IR) were improved by carnitine supplementation. Modulating the intramitochondrial acetyl-CoA/CoA ratio and the activity of the PDH complex, as described above, are explained in the paper as important mechanisms behind impacts of carnitine supplementation. These beneficial effects of carnitine supplementation led the authors to the conclusion that carnitine might be an effective tool for improving glucose tolerance in insulin resistant states. Insulin resistance of the dairy cow at the start of lactation is well known and repeatedly described in the literature (Sinclair, 2010; Martens, 2013).

Carnitine and inflammation

Inflammation may impair carnitine biosynthesis and carnitine uptake into the cell (Eder, 2013). Research shows that subclinical and chronic inflammation in the transition period of farm animals is an emerging serious problem. Trevisi, Amadori, Archetti, Lacetera and Bertoni (2011) concluded that inflammatory phenomena of varying seriousness in the transition period of dairy cows may aggravate negative energy balance due to lower dry matter intake and/or waste of energy and nutrients. That inflammation and energy metabolism are closely linked is explained by Liu, Brown, Gazzar, McPhail, Millet, Rao, Vachharajani, Yoza and McGall (2012), revealing that the initiating pro-inflammatory phase of acute and chronic inflammation is anabolic and needs glucose as the primary fuel, whereas the opposing adaption phase is catabolic requiring fatty acid oxidation. This is in accordance with the transition period of farm animals shifting from anabolic to catabolic at parturition. Ye and Keller (2011) described the regulation of energy metabolism by inflammation as a feedback response of the body to get rid of the energy surplus stored in body fat, with a reverse of these chronic inflammatory events under energy restriction. Steinberg, Watt and Febbraio (2009) illustrated how

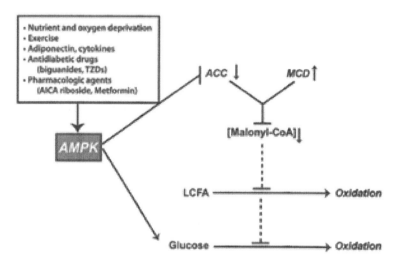

Figure 4. AMPK stimulation of glucose and fatty acid oxidation (Hue and Taegtmeyer, 2009).

energy metabolism is steered by inflammatory agents, for example the cytokines TNF-α, IL-6, resistin. The enzyme adenosine monophosphate-activated protein kinase (AMPK) is impacted by Inflammation (Hue *et al.* 2009; Steinberg *et al.*, 2009). Towler and Hardie (2007) see the enzyme playing a key role in maintaining energy balance at the whole body level. According to Zhang, Zhou and Li (2009) AMPK controls glucose homeostasis through inhibition of gluconeogenic gene expression and hepatic glucose production. Locher, Rehage, Khraim, Meyer, Dänicke, Hansen and Huber (2012) showed that lipolysis in early lactation of dairy cows is associated with an increase in phosphorylation of AMPK and the ratio of pAMPK/AMPK in bovine adipose tissues. AMPK stimulates glucose and fatty acid utilization. Activation of AMPK leads to acetyl-CoA carboxylase (ACC) inactivation, possibly together with malonyl-CoA decarboxylase (MCD) activation, which decreases malonyl-CoA concentration. Malonyl-CoA works as an inhibitor for the fatty acid shuttle into the mitochondria. Decrease of Malonyl-CoA concentration hence favours fatty acid oxidation by accelerating transport of fatty acids to β-oxidation (Hue and Taegtmeyer, 2009).

These findings should give reason to investigate further if inflammation not only worsens, but probably even triggers negative energy balance, or at least acts as the driver in a vicious circle. Inhibition of carnitine biosynthesis and carnitine uptake into cells due to inflammation probably aggravates the problem, as shown in Figure 5, due to the fact that "blocking the entrance to open the gate" is more or less reversed.

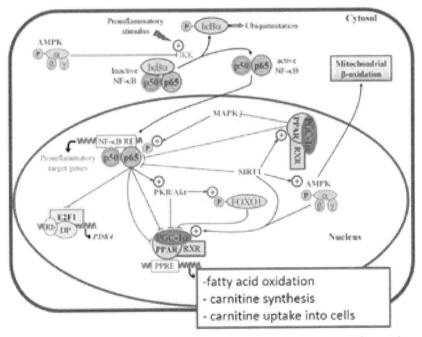

Figure 5. Inflammation impairs PPAR-regulated fatty acid oxidation, carnitine synthesis and carnitine uptake into cells (Palomer, 2013, adapted by Eder, 2013).

Carnitine in dairy cows

It is well known that energy balance of modern high genetic merit dairy cows is negative after parturition. Extent and duration of negative energy balance in early lactation has been increased by genetic selection of cows for initial and rapid increase to peak milk yield. Many health risks are correlated with negative energy balance (Martens, 2013), listed in table 2.

Table 2: Incidence rate of metabolic disorders in early lactation in a field study including 5,884 cows in 528 farms in 10 European countries (Suthar, Raposo, Deniz, and Heuwieser, 2012 in Martens, 2013)

Metabolic disorder	Mean	Minimum	Maximum
Retained placenta	10.4	5.7	28.1
Milk fever	4.0	0	9.5
Metritis	9.6	3.2	24.9
Mastitis	6.1	1.8	29.9
Subclinical ketosis	21.5	11.2	36.6
Clinical ketosis	3.7	0.7	11.1
Laminitis	3.3	1.2	10.4
Displaced abomasum	2.7	0.4	8.9

To cover this lack of energy in early lactation cows mobilize body fat, leading to an increasing quantity of acetyl-CoA in the mitochondria in accordance with the physiological mechanisms explained above. At some point the quantity of acetyl-CoA will exceed the capacity of β-oxidation. In ruminants the situation is aggravated due to a lack of oxaloacetate which is needed for gluconeogenesis. Consequently ketogenesis accelerates. More and more ketone bodies are built up, resulting in subclinical or even clinical ketosis (Jeroch, Drochner and Simon, 2008). In a field study 39% of the cows in 131 herds in 5 European countries were classified as having ketosis (Berge and Vertenten, 2014). Considering the role of carnitine in modulating the acetyl-CoA/CoA ratio it is self-evident to explore the physiological role of carnitine in dairy cows in the transition period. Schlegel, Keller, Hirche, Geißler, Schwarz, Ringseis, Stangl and Eder (2012) investigated the effect of lactation on carnitine metabolism of dairy cows. They showed that the loss of carnitine via milk in early lactation of dairy cows was 215.5 mmol/l in week 1. By week 14, carnitine content in milk had decreased to 101.5 mmol/l. It is noteworthy that the ratio free carnitine/acetyl carnitine was inverted from 84.5/131.1 to 60.2/41.3. These relations correspond with the carnitine blood parameters which were analyzed concurrently. Fürll and Harmeyer (1997) found similar results. The reversed acetyl-carnitine/carnitine ratio in milk and blood can be considered as a consequence of the modulation of the acetyl-CoA/CoA ratio in the mitochondria. Moreover the study showed for the first time that hepatic mRNA abundances of genes involved in carnitine synthesis and cellular uptake of carnitine in dairy cows are increased during the transition from late pregnancy to early lactation. According to the metabolic parameters in the blood and in liver biopsy, non-esterified fatty acids (NEFA), triglycerides and BHB, however, the cows in this experiment obviously could cope with the negative energy balance. Considering that carnitine biosynthesis and uptake into the cell are increased, while carnitine concentration in blood, total carnitine and particularly free carnitine, are reduced, Eder (2013) suggested a need for additional exogenous carnitine in the transition period to complement endogenous biosynthesis. Finally, in view of the studies and trials revealing positive effects of carnitine supplementation, the authors suspect that carnitine might be the rate-limiting factor of hepatic β-oxidation. Carlson, McFadden, D'Angelo, Woodworth and Drackley (2007) investigated the effects of dietary carnitine supplementation on liver lipid accumulation, hepatic nutrient metabolism, and lactation in multiparous cows during the periparturient period. The quantities of carnitine supplied were 6 g/d, 50 g/d, and 100 g/d in the form of non-rumen-protected carnitine. All carnitine treatments decreased liver total lipid triacylglycerol (TG) accumulation, increased glycogen and thereby improved TG/glycogen ratio in the liver significantly on day 10 after calving. The authors thus conclude that by decreasing liver lipid accumulation and stimulating hepatic glucose output, carnitine might improve glucose status and diminish the risk of developing metabolic disorders during early lactation. In a field trial, Scholz, Ahrens, Menn and von Heimendahl (2014) divided 262 Holstein-Friesian dairy cattle into two groups according to their lactation number. The trial group (CP) received 10 g/d of a rumen-protected carnitine product i.e. 2 g/d pure carnitine per cow and day. The control group (C) was fed 10 g/d barley instead. There was no significant impact on crucial blood parameters within the physiological range indicating that the metabolic stress of the herd was not critical. Nevertheless, carnitine lowered the content of NEFA in the blood by trend, improved fat/protein ratio in milk and reduced milk somatic cell count. Significantly more cows were pregnant at day 200 of lactation due to carnitine supplementation. Moreover, carnitine improved the health status and fertility of the cows proved by a significant decline in the number of veterinary treatments (Table 3).

Table 3: Impact of carnitine on fertility and veterinary treatments (Scholz *et al*, 2014)

	Control group	Carnitine group
Days open	75	74
Insemination ratio	2.3	1.9
Pregnancy rate[*]	71[a]	86[b]
Total treatments	1.64[a]	1.17[c]
Fertility treatments	0.28[a]	0.17[c]
Udder treatments	1.32[a]	0.93[c]

* % pregnant cows at day > 200, cows not pregnant were culled; a, b significant difference between groups.

Carnitine and fertility

A detailed understanding of the mechanisms of insulin action, insulin resistance and hyperinsulinaemia in cattle is lacking, in contrast to humans and rodents. However, mechanisms of insulin action in ruminants are believed to be similar to those of other species. Hyperinsulinaemia in cattle is associated with impaired oocyte quality and embryo development (Sinclair, 2010). Diskin, Murphy and Sreenan (2006) showed changes in the reproductive outcome of British-Friesian in 2006 compared to 1980. Losses due to early embryo death increased from 28% to 43% while trouble-free calving dropped from 55% to 40%. Fertilisation error and late embryo death remained constant at 10% and 7%, respectively. Wade and Jones (2004) developed a working hypothesis to explain the link between the physiological controls of energy balance and fertility, as a result of natural selection such that reproduction is deferred during lean times, particularly in female mammals. Martens (2012) refers to this working hypothesis in his essay on energy metabolism and fertility of the cow, and moreover supports it by referencing corresponding results from sheep and cattle. It is hypothesised that a so called "fuel detector" (energy sensor) in the hindbrain detects oxidisable metabolic fuels in the blood, probably mainly glucose. If sufficient glucose for oxidation is available a neuronal signal is transmitted to the forebrain to release GnRH. A lack of these oxidisable fuels, e.g. during fasting, excessive energy expenditure, or diabetes mellitus, can inhibit both GnRH release and oestrous behaviour. Disruption of the signal cascade by cutting the nerve in small rodents allows normal reproduction and oestrous behaviour to proceed under negative energy balance. This confirms the working hypothesis mentioned above (Wade and Jones, 2004; Martens, 2012). By improving insulin resistance and glucose tolerance accompanied by increased hepatic glucose output as described previously, carnitine provides a promising tool to improve reproductive performance in dairy cows. Nevertheless, more research is necessary to further elucidate and confirm these metabolic mechanisms.

Conclusion

Physiological functions of carnitine are manifold. Biosynthesis is reduced under anabolic conditions, e.g. in pregnancy. Carnitine demand is increased in catabolic metabolism such as negative energy balance after parturition. Subclinical and chronic inflammation may aggravate the problem by impairing energy metabolism and by inhibiting carnitine biosynthesis. Exogenous carnitine reduces insulin resistance and improves glucose tolerance in humans and monogastric animals. Consequently, it would seem appropriate to supply additional exogenous carnitine to dairy cows in the transition period to limit the risk of metabolic disorders due to carnitine deficiency occurring during pregnancy and body fat mobilization in early lactation.

Nevertheless, detailed knowledge of the physiological role of carnitine in dairy cows, and also regarding the impact of inflammation on energy metabolism, is still scarce requiring further research for elucidation.

Acknowledgements

I would like to express my gratitude to Prof. Klaus Eder, University Gießen, Germany, for critical discussion of the manuscript. In addition I would like to express my appreciation to my colleagues Lorraine Herfort and David Beaumont for proofreading the manuscript.

References

Berge, A.C. and Vertenten, G. (2014) A field study to determine the prevalence, dairy herd management systems, and fresh cow clinical conditions associated with ketosis in western European dairy herds. *Journal of Dairy Science, 97*, 2145-2154.

Carlson, D.B., McFadden, J.W., D'Angelo, A.D., Woodworth, J.C. and Drackley, J.K. (2007) Dietary L-Carnitine Affects Periparturient Nutrient Metabolism and Lactation in Multiparous Cows. *Journal of Dairy Science, 90*, 3422-3441.

Diskin, M.G., Murphy, J.J. and Sreenan, J.M. (2006) Embryo survival in dairy cows managed under pastoral conditions. *Animal Reproduction Science, 96*, 297-311.

Eder, K. (2009) Review Article - Influence of L-carnitine on metabolism and performance of sows. *British Journal of Nutrition, 102*, 645–654.

Eder, K. (2013) The physiological role of carnitine, *presentation Lohmann in Hamburg, Dec. 12th*.

Flanagan, J.L. Simmons, P.A., Vehige, J., Willcox, M.D.P. and Garret, Q. (2010) Role of carnitine in disease – Review. *Nutrition and Metabolism, 7:30*, 2-14. (http://www.nutritionandmetabolism.com/content/7/1/30)

Fuerll, M and Harmeyer, J. C. (1997) Carnitin-Konzentrationen im Blut bei Hochleistungskühen im peripartalen Zeitraum. In Schubert R, Flachowski G, Bitsch R, Jahreis G. (Eds.) *Vitamine und Zusatzstoffe in der Ernährung von Mensch und Tier*. Verlag Buch- und Kunstdruckerei Keßler GmbH, Jena, 297-303, ISBN 3-00-002381-X

Harmeyer, J. and Schlumborn, C. (1997) Die physiologische Bedeutung von L-Carnitin und Effekte von Carnitinzulagen bei Haustieren, in *Proc. 6th. Symp. Vitamine u. weitere Zusatzstoffe bei Mensch und Tier.*

Hue, L. and Taegtmeyer, H. (2009) The randle cycle revisited: a new head for an old hat. *AJP Endocrinological Metabolism, 297*, E578-E591

Jeroch, H., Drochner, W. and Simon, O. (2008) *Ernährung landwirtschaftlicher Nutztiere,* Verlag Eugen Ulmer, 2nd edition, p 443.

Locher, L.F., Rehage, J., Khraim, N., Meyer,U., Dänicke, S., Hansen, K. and Huber, K. (2012) Lipolysis in early lactation is associated with an increase in phosphorylation of adenosine monophosphate-activated kinase (AMPK)α1 in adipose tissue of dairy cows. *Journal of Dairy Science,* **95,** 2497-2504,

Luppa, D. (2004) Beteiligung von L-Carnitin an der Regulation des Fett- und Kohlenhydratstoffwechsels. *Klinische Sportmedizin / Clinical Sports Medicine (KCS),* **5**(1), 25 – 34.

Liu, T.F., Brown, C.M., Gazzar, M., McPhail, L., Millet, P., Rao, A., Vachhrajani, V.T., Yoza, B.K. and McCall, C. E. (2012) Fueling the flame: Bioenergy couples metabolism and inflammation. *Journal of Leukocyte Biology,* **92,** 499-507.

Martens, H. (2012) Energiestoffwechsel und Fruchtbarkeit der Kuh. *Tierärztliche Umschau,* **67,** 496-503.

Martens, H. (2013) Erkrankungen von Milchkühen in der frühen Laktationsphase – Risikofaktor negative Energiebilanz und Hyperketonämie. *Tierärztliche Umschau,* **68,** 463-476.

Palomer, X, Salvado, L., Barroso, E. and Vazques-Carrera, M. (2013) An overview of the crosstalk and metabolic dysregulation during diabetic cardiomyopathy *International Journal of Cardiology* , **168,** 3160-3172.

Randle, P.J., Garland, P.B., Hales, C.N. and Newsholme, E.A. (1963) The Glucose Fatty-Acid Cycle Its Role In Insulin Sensitivity And Metabolic Disturbances Of Diabetes Mellitus. *The Lancet,* **281,** 785-789.

Ringseis, R., Hanisch, N., Seliger, G. and Eder, K. (2010) Low availability of carnitine precursors as a possible reason for the diminished plasma carnitine concentrations in pregnant women. *BioMedCentral, Pregnancy and childbirth,* **10,** 17. (http://www.biomedcentral.com/1471-2393/10/17)

Ringseis, R., Keller, J. and Eder, K. (2012) Role of carnitine in the regulation of glucose homeostasis and insulin sensitivity: Evidence from in vivo and in vitro studies with carnitine supplementation and carnitine deficiency. *European Journal of Nutrition,* **51,** 1-18.

Schlegel, G., Keller, J., Hirche, F., Geißler, F., Schwarz, F.J., Ringseis, R., Stangl, G.I. and Eder, K. (2012) Expression of genes involved in hepatic carnitine synthesis and uptake in dairy cows in the transition period and at different stages of lactation. *BioMedCentral, Veterinary Research,* **8,** 28 (http://www.biomedcentral.com/1746-6148/8/28)

Scholz, H., Ahrens, A., Menn, F. and Heimendahl, E.v. (2014) Einsatz von pansengeschütztem L-Carnitin bei Milchkühen in der Vorbereitungs- und der Hochleistungsphase. *Züchtungskunde,* **86,** 115-122.

Schrauwen, P., Timmers, S. and Hesselink, K.C. (2013): Blocking the entrance to open the gate. *Diabetes,* **62,** 703-705.

Sinclair, K. (2010) Declining fertility, insulin resistance and fatty acid metabolism in dairy cows: Developmental consequences for the oocyte and pre-implantation embryo. *Acta Scientiae Veterinariae,* **38(Supl 2),** 545-557.

Steinberg, G.R., Watt, M.J. and Febbraio, M.A. (2009) Cytokine regulation of AMPK signalling. *Frontiers Bioscience,* **14,** 1902-1916.

Towler, M.C. and Hardie, D.G. (2007) AMP-activated Protein Kinase in Metabolic Control and Insulin Signaling. *Circulation Reasearch,* **100**, 328-341.

Trevisi, E., Amadori, M., Archetti, I., Lacetera, N. and Bertoni, G. (2011) Inflammatory Response and Acute Phase Proteins in the Transition Period of High-Yielding Dairy Cows. In *Acute Phase Proteins as Early Non-Specific Biomarkers of Human and Veterinary Diseases* (Ed, Francisco Veas), ISBN: 978-953-307-873-1, pp 355-380.

Vaz, F.M. and Wanders, R.J.A. (2002) Review article: Carnitine biosynthesis in mammals. *Biochemical Society Journal,* **361**, 417-429.

Wade, G.N. and Jones, J.E. (2004) Neuroendocrinology of nutritional infertility. *American journal of physiology. Regulatory, integrative and comparative physiology,* **287**, R1277-R1296.

Wüsten, O. (1999) Insulinresistenz im Postprandialen Lipidstoffwechsel bei Metabolischem Syndrom – Untersuchungen zur Glukosetoleranz nach oraler Fettaufnahme. *Inaugural Dissertation Medizin Univ. Gießen.*

Ye, J. and Keller, J.N. (2010) Regulation of energy metabolism by inflammation: A feedback response in obesity and calorie restriction, *Aging,* **2 No.6**, 361-368

Zhang, B., Zhou, G. and Li, C. (2009) AMPK: An Emerging Drug Target for Diabetes and Metabolic Syndrome. *Cell Metabolism,* **9,** 407- 416.

3

Considerations for Feeding Starch to High-Yielding Dairy Cows

C. K. REYNOLDS*, D. J. HUMPHRIES*, A. M. VAN VUUREN†,
J. DIJKSTRA‡, AND A. BANNINK†.

Centre for Dairy Research, University of Reading, P.O. Box 237, Earley Gate, Reading, RG6 6AR, UK.

†Wageningen UR Livestock Research, P.O. Box 338, 6700 AH Wageningen, the Netherlands.

‡Animal Nutrition Group, Wageningen University, P.O. Box 338, 6700 AH Wageningen, the Netherlands

Introduction

There has long been interest in the potential benefits and risks of feeding starch to lactating dairy cows (e.g. Henderson and Reaves, 1954; Armsby, 1922) and there have been numerous reviews published on the utilization of starch by ruminants for production (e.g. Waldo, 1973; Owens *et al.*, 1986; Nocek and Tamminga, 1991; Huntington, 1997; Firkins *et al.*, 2001). In a previous publication for the 31st University of Nottingham Feed Manufacturers Conference the effects of feeding starch to lactating dairy cows on nutrient availability and milk production and composition were reviewed, including the effects of altering site of starch digestion within the digestive tract (Reynolds *et al.*, 1997). In recent years there has continued to be research into effects of starch type and site of starch digestion on production and metabolism of lactating dairy cows (e.g. Reynolds, 2006), along with a pervasive concern over the potential negative effects of sub-acute ruminal acidosis (SARA), the future demand for food for a growing human population, and the ethics of feeding starch to ruminants. Our objective is to revisit key points raised in these previous reviews in light of more recent research, the sustained increase in milk yield and nutrient requirements of lactating dairy cows, and concerns regarding the future role of ruminants in sustainable food production systems.

Why feed starch to dairy cows?

Dairy farmers are paid for the amount and quality of the milk they sell, which has been incentive for increasing milk yield per cow through genetic selection and advances in feeding and farm management. The increase in average annual milk yield per cow has continued year on year for 70 years in the USA (www.usda.gov/nass) and has been particularly evident in the Holstein breed, which represents the majority of the current dairy cow population in many countries (e.g. USA, http://www.epa.gov/oecaagct/ag101/dairysystems.html). The capacity of the dairy cow for feed intake has increased along with milk yield, but body energy loss in early lactation appears to be an unavoidable consequence of high milk energy output as increases in milk energy output typically precede increases in net energy intake (Reynolds, 2005). Indeed, the high feed dry matter intake (DMI) of modern dairy cows is in part a consequence of the effects of the large nutrient requirements for milk synthesis on appetite and body energy deficit (Allen *et al.*, 2005). However, excessive body fat mobilization can have negative metabolic consequences (Ingvarsten and Anderson, 2000), including negative effects on health, reproduction, and longevity (Grummer, 1993). To meet nutrient requirements of high-yielding dairy cows nutritionists will typically formulate diets for maximal intake of absorbable nutrients and metabolisable energy (ME) using available feed resources. Diet digestibility has a major impact on nutrient supply both in terms of ME content and the limitation imposed on DMI by rumen fill (Zom *et al.*, 2012). In practical terms, an increase in diet digestibility and nutrient intake has often been realized through the addition of more rapidly-digestible concentrate feeds containing starch from cereal grains. Dairy cow rations are formulated on the basis of concentrations and characteristics of carbohydrates, fats, and proteins (as well as minerals and vitamins). Whilst there have historically been a number of analytical approaches used to characterize the chemical composition of feeds, the most common approach currently is for the carbohydrate fractions to be characterized by determining neutral detergent fibre (NDF) concentration and then calculating the neutral detergent solubles or non-NDF carbohydrates (non-fibre carbohydrates or NFC) by difference calculation. The NFC fraction includes starch, sugars, and pectin, which also can be measured individually, but the starch component is often the largest fraction of the NFC in diets traditionally fed to high yielding dairy cows. That said it is important to realize that concentrations of NFC are not solely starch when interpreting effects of diet composition reported in the scientific literature. In the case of legumes a large portion of NFC are present as pectin, which are soluble in neutral detergent solution (Cassida *et al.*, 2007). The NDF includes the 'plant cell walls' including hemicellulose, cellulose, lignin, and cutin. The NDF concentration of the diet is important in terms of effects on rate and extent of digestion, rumen fill, and DMI capacity, as well as effects on rumen health. In simple terms, specific recommendations are given for NDF and NFC concentrations in rations that will allow maximal intake of digestible, rumen fermentable substrates without negative effects of excess fermentation end products and acid accumulation (e.g. NRC, 2001). These recommendations are then adjusted for specific sources of NDF and NFC, with the concentration of 'physically effective NDF' (peNDF) of particular importance for effects on rumination and rumen health (e.g. Weiss, 2002).

Site of starch digestion

As a consequence of extensive carbohydrate fermentation in the rumen ruminants normally absorb little if any glucose from their small intestine and must rely on glucose synthesis from propionate and other precursors to meet their glucose requirements, which are substantial in high-yielding dairy cows. Dairy cows derive the majority of their ME and metabolisable protein (MP) from rumen microbial production of volatile fatty acids (VFA; largely acetate, propionate, and n-butyrate) and protein, respectively. Propionate from rumen fermentation is the major glucose precursor along with lactate, glucogenic amino acids, i-butyrate and n-valerate. Increased ruminal digestion of starch will generally shift VFA patterns in the rumen towards a higher ratio of propionate (glucogenic) to acetate and n-butyrate (Bannink *et al.*, 2006), which are used for fat synthesis in mammary and other tissues (lipogenic).

Rate of starch degradation is determined by a number of factors, including starch type, maturity, processing, and rate of passage through the digestive tract. For the more widely available starch sources, rate of ruminal degradation is faster and digestibility is higher for wheat and barley and lower for maize and sorghum starches, with oat starch intermediate (Firkins *et al.*, 2001; Larsen *et al.*, 2009). In addition, peas and beans are another potential starch source in Northern European diets. Legume starch was found to have a lower rate of ruminal degradation, but also a very limited digestibility in the small intestine in lactating dairy cows (Larsen *et al.*, 2009). Cereal grains must be processed to make starch granules accessible for microbial fermentation in the rumen or hindgut or enzymatic digestion in the small intestine and processing method has a major effect on site and extent of starch digestion (Firkins *et al.*, 2001; Larsen *et al.*, 2009). Steam flaking is one processing method that markedly improves the digestibility of maize and sorghum starch, which is inherently more resistant to rumen and total digestion (Theuer *et al.*, 1999). Larsen *et al.* (2009) compared the site and extent of starch digestion from various sources available in Northern Europe and found that grinding greatly increased starch digestibility compared to rolling. Rolling was associated with a larger particle size, which reduced accessibility of enzymes and limited starch digestion in the small intestine. In this regard rate of passage may also be an important factor for starch digestibility in the small intestine (and hindgut). Without the application of novel technologies to protect highly digestible starch from ruminal degradation without limiting digestibility in the small intestine (Deckardt *et al.*, 2013), starch sources that are associated with greater rumen outflow of starch to the small intestine are inherently less digestible in the small intestine (Nocek and Tamminga, 1991), such that an increasing proportion of postruminal starch digestion occurs in the large intestine or cecum as postruminal starch flow increases (Reynolds, 2006; Larsen *et al.*, 2009). Microbial fermentation of starch in the hindgut will provide VFA for absorption, but microbial protein produced will not be available to the animal and will increase faecal nitrogen. Excessive starch fermentation in the hindgut may have negative effects in terms of fibre digestion and absorption of microbial lipopolysaccharide (Gressley *et al.*, 2011; Li *et al.*, 2012). In addition, starch digestion in the hindgut also may have negative effects on NDF digestion. In dairy cows greater starch flow to the hindgut (1.39 vs 0.32 kg) with higher dietary starch inclusion was associated with less NDF digestion (0 vs 12 g/kg inflow; van Vuuren *et al.*, 2010).

Another processing method for cereal grains that has been used extensively for wheat (and other cereals) is treatment with sodium hydroxide (Phipps *et al.*, 2001). Sodium hydroxide treated wheat is less degradable in the rumen than ground wheat, which increases rate of ruminal starch outflow, yet the starch is still digestible in the small intestine such that a lower proportion of the starch reaching the small intestine is fermented in the hindgut (Larsen *et al.*, 2009). It is important to remember that a major source of starch in rations for high yielding dairy cows in many regions is forage maize silage. As maize silage starch is less mature than maize harvested for grain, maize silage starch digestibility is higher than for maize meal starch in both the rumen and small intestine (Moharrery *et al.*, 2014).

The total digestive tract digestibility of dietary starch in lactating dairy cows is high and typically greater than 85 % for cereal starch unless grain processing is insufficient for exposure of starch granules to enzymatic digestion (Firkins *et al.*, 2001; Reynolds, 2006; Larsen *et al.*, 2009; Moharrery *et al.*, 2014). Measurement of site of starch digestion within the digestive tract of dairy cows has been obtained using gut cannulation techniques that allow measurement of passage of digesta at key sites (e.g. the omasum, duodenum, or ileum). Digestion in the rumen varies with starch source and other factors as discussed previously, with digestion of more than 6 kg/d reported (Figure 1; Reynolds, 2006). Unlike dietary fibre, rumen starch fermentation does not appear to be reduced by acid accumulation at higher rates of intake and fermentation (Oba and Allen, 2003). The capacity for total starch digestion in the postruminal tract is also high, with postruminal digestion of over 5 kg/d reported and no evidence of a limit at higher rates of rumen outflow (Reynolds *et al.*, 1997; Reynolds, 2006). Total postruminal digestion includes digestion in both the small intestine and hindgut (large intestine and cecum), and the extent to which total postruminal digestion occurs in the small intestine varies across studies. Measurements of small intestinal digestion are less available than measurements of postruminal digestion (duodenal flow minus faecal excretion) due to inherent difficulties in the techniques required, but digestion of up to 2.5 kg/d of starch in the small intestine of lactating dairy cows has been reported (Figure 2; Reynolds, 2006). Starch reaching the hindgut is less digestible as it has escaped digestion in the upper tract, but digestion of as much as 1.7 kg/d has been reported for the hindgut of lactating dairy cows fed large amounts of maize meal (Knowlton *et al.*, 1998). In non-lactating cattle there is evidence that as starch flow to the small intestine increases starch digestibility decreases (Matthe *et al.*, 2001; Moharrery *et al.*, 2014) and a declining digestibility of starch in the small intestine of lactating dairy cows is also evident at higher duodenal starch flows (Figure 3; Reynolds, 2006).

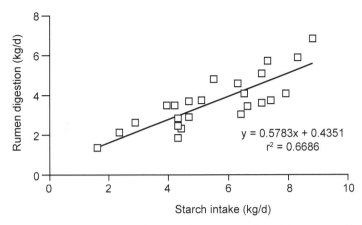

Figure 1. Ruminal starch digestion in lactating dairy cows. Adapted from Reynolds (2006).

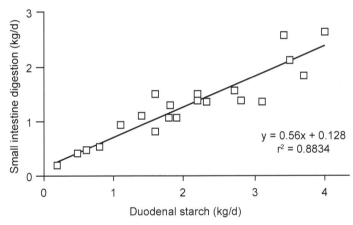

Figure 2. Starch digestion in the small intestine of lactating dairy cows. Adapted from Reynolds (2006).

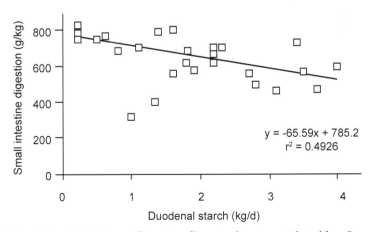

Figure 3. Starch digestibility in the small intestine of lactating dairy cows. Adapted from Reynolds (2006).

However, differences in starch type and structure associated with reduced ruminal digestion may also have contributed to the decrease in apparent starch digestibility in the small intestine observed with increasing flow into the duodenum.

Predicting the rate and extent of starch digestion in the rumen is essential for predictions of ME and MP supply using numerous feed evaluation systems. Fractional rate of starch digestion is most commonly estimated using the *in situ* technique where samples are incubated in the rumen of a 'representative' animal within nylon bags and the disappearance of starch from the bags over time is measured. These estimates of rate of digestion are combined with estimates of fractional rate of passage out of the rumen to estimate rate of starch degradation in the rumen. Major concerns with this technique are the loss of starch from the bags due to simple washout, how to measure or estimate the fractional rate of passage of particulate starch, and how to estimate effective rates of degradation and passage of the 'washout' fraction. An alternative approach used is the *in vitro* gas production technique where rate of gas production and disappearance of starch are indicative of rate and extent of digestion. However, in this case the rate of gas production reflects fermentation of the organic matter present, not solely the starch fraction. As for the *in situ* procedure, calculation of ruminal degradation rate using gas production kinetics in vitro requires an estimate of fractional passage rate from the rumen. Extent of digestion can also be measured using cannulated cattle, which is expensive and laborious. Significant relationships with *in vivo* ruminal starch degradability have been found for both *in situ* and *in vitro* approaches (Weisbjerg *et al.*, 2011), but there was a stronger correlation for *in situ* estimates (r = 0.84 vs r = 0.76). In addition, they found that fractional degradation rates (k_d) based on *in situ* estimates were unrealistic for some starch sources. Hindle *et al.* (2005) compared *in vivo*, *in situ* and *in vitro* measurements of site and extent of digestion of 3 starch sources using lactating dairy cows. They found that predictions of effective ruminal degradability based on *in situ* degradability may under predict ruminal degradation, and therefore over predict rumen outflow, and thus refinements to estimates using both techniques were needed. Hindle *et al.* (2005) suggested that animals used for *in situ* or *in vitro* rumen incubations should be adapted to the starch sources evaluated as using a rumen with a microbial population that is not adapted to the starch and feed matrix evaluated could lead to an underestimation of ruminal degradability. Ultimately estimates of true rates of ruminal starch degradation will require better representation of the dynamic nature of feed starch and rumen microbial interactions, as well as the contributions of protozoa and microbial starch to ruminal starch degradation *in vivo*. Similar concerns must also be addressed in order to estimate rates of digestion and degradation of starch in the small intestine and hindgut. In addition, the relationship between rate of starch degradation and ruminal retention time requires further attention.

Benefits of feeding starch

Benefits of feeding starch include increased ME and MP supply and thus greater milk and milk protein yield compared to feeding less digestible NDF. These benefits are attributable to the increased digestible energy (DE), decreased methane emission (see below), and thus ME concentration of starch compared to fibrous components of the diet as well as the higher DMI of starchy feeds. The benefits of the increased nutritional supply from feeding grains for milk yield have long been recognized (e.g. Henderson and Reaves, 1954; Armsby, 1922), as well as the potential positive effects of feeding starch on milk protein concentration and yield through effects on ruminal microbial protein synthesis and metabolic effects of increased propionate or glucose absorption (Reynolds, 2006; Rigout *et al.*, 2003). Although at *ad libitum* intakes feeding concentrates will reduce total forage intake, the net effect is typically an increase in DMI and ME supply for production, unless starch fermentation inhibits fibre digestion excessively (Reynolds *et al.*, 1997).

Effects on methane yield

In recent years there has been much concern regarding methane emissions from ruminants and options for reducing them. There is no question that ruminant farm animals produce methane as a consequence of ruminal microbial activity in their gastrointestinal tract and that their methane emission accounts for a substantial portion of global methane emission inventory (http://faostat3.fao.org/faostat-gateway/go/to/download/G1/*/E). The methane emitted by dairy cows is primarily produced by rumen archeae through the reduction of CO_2, which provides a route of disposal for H_2 arising from ruminal fermentation. As governments have committed to future reductions in greenhouse gas emissions, there is pressure to reduce methane emissions attributable to agriculture that has led to an explosion of research activity into feeding and management options or technologies to limit methane emissions by ruminant livestock. This is not a new area of research. As methane accounts for on average 6.5% of total energy consumption in dairy cows, or about 600 L per day for a lactating dairy cow, there has long been research interest in approaches to reduce this 'waste' of energy. An early summary of measurements of methane emissions from cattle obtained during energy metabolism studies showed that there was a positive relationship between intake of digestible carbohydrate and methane emission (Bratzler an Forbes, 1940). However, as early as 1907 Kellner reported the amount of methane produced was lower for digested starch than for digested straw (Washburn and Brody, 1937). More recent meta-analysis of published data and experimental observations have reported that in addition to the amount of feed DMI, the methane produced per unit DMI (methane yield) is affected by the proportions of starch and fibre in the diet consumed, with methane yield reduced with increased starch concentration. In this regard Mills *et al.* (2003) found that the ratio of starch to acid detergent fibre (ADF; cellulose and lignin) was related to methane yield, whilst more recent studies have reported that methane production of lactating dairy cows was related to NDF intake (Aguerre *et al.*, 2011). In another analysis of data available from energy balance studies, the effects of starch on methane yield plateaued at higher concentrations in diets fed to growing beef cattle (Mills *et al.*, 2009), whilst Hristov *et al.* (2013) concluded that inclusion of starch-rich concentrates was more effective in reducing methane yield when diet concentrate levels are greater than 35 to 40%. In lactating dairy cows fed diets formulated to contain varying proportions of maize and grass silage but equal amounts of starch and NDF, methane yield was higher for the high grass silage diets (Reynolds *et al.*, 2010). This suggests that in addition to starch and NDF or ADF concentrations, the type of carbohydrate (starch, sugars, hemicellulose, cellulose, etc.) and rate and extent of degradation are also factors affecting methane yield.

Effects of starch versus fibre on methane yield are attributable to patterns of ruminal fermentation, with higher rates of starch fermentation associated with a shift towards more propionate and less acetate and n-butyrate, which is more glucogenic through the provision of propionate for glucose synthesis in the liver. In contrast, higher fibre diets are more lipogenic through the provision of greater proportions of acetate and n-butyrate which are used for fatty acid synthesis in the mammary gland. Whereas synthesis of propionate provides a 'sink' for H_2, reducing the availability of excess H_2 for methane production, synthesis of acetate and n-butyrate is a 'source' of H_2.

Effects of feeding starch on energy supply in early lactation

Another purported benefit of feeding starch in early lactation is the potential positive effects of increased ME and/or glucogenic nutrient supply on body energy balance and reproduction. As mentioned previously, excessive body energy loss in early lactation is a concern for high yielding dairy cows for a number or reasons. Excessive body fat mobilization in early lactation can contribute to the development of metabolic disorders, including fatty liver and ketosis, and is associated with shifts in hormonal status that are linked to reduced fertility (Grummer, 1993; Butler, 2000). Therefore, an approach often taken with diets for high yielding dairy cows in the early postpartum period has been to increase the energy concentration of the diet through added starch or fat. Potential benefits of feeding starch in addition to a greater supply of ME and net energy for lactation (NE_l) include a greater supply of glucose for milk lactose synthesis. Glucose supply for milk synthesis is substantial and greater than milk lactose secretion due to glucose requirements of the mammary gland and other body tissues and can amount to over 3 kg/d for a cow producing 40 kg of milk (Reynolds *et al.*, 2003). A common assumption is that milk yield in early lactation is limited by glucose and glucogenic precursor supply and that one benefit of feeding starch in early lactation is an increased milk yield through increased provision of propionate, the predominate glucose precursor, or glucose absorption from starch that reaches the small intestine. Similarly, it is dogma that glucose synthesis in early lactation requires a greater contribution from amino acids such that the demand for glucose through synthesis in the liver limits milk protein concentration and yield. Thus it is generally believed that feeding starch will benefit milk and milk protein yield of the early lactation cow through greater absorption of propionate from the rumen and/or glucose from the small intestine, increased total glucose supply, and reduced reliance on amino acids for glucose synthesis.

As reviewed previously (Reynolds, 2006), in previous studies where site of sorghum starch digestion has been altered by steam flaking, which increased ruminal degradability, milk yield and protein concentration were higher when a greater proportion of starch was digested in the rumen (Theuer et al., 1999). This reflected a greater fermentable energy supply to the rumen, but also a greater total tract starch digestibility and thus NE_l supply. In studies where propionate has been incrementally infused into the rumen or glucose incrementally infused into the abomasum or duodenum of lactating dairy cows, there was a curvilinear increase in milk yield, a linear increase in milk protein concentration, and a curvilinear decrease in milk fat concentration (Rigout et al., 2003). In these studies glucose was infused postruminally as a proxy for increased glucose absorption from starch digestion in the small intestine. However, the metabolic response to glucose infused into the abomasum or duodenum may differ from the response to increased starch supply to the small intestine because the endocrine responses to glucose absorption in the duodenum may differ from the responses to glucose absorption from the jejunum or ileum where glucose will be liberated from starch digestion (Reynolds, 2006).

Early data from sheep showed that it is energetically more efficient to digest starch directly to absorbable glucose in the small intestine, rather than digesting the starch in the rumen to VFA and other products, of which the propionate can be converted to glucose in the liver (Armstrong et al., 1960). For this reason there has long been interest in the potential benefits of "rumen escape" starch for high-yielding dairy cows, particularly during early lactation when glucose requirements are high relative to ME intake. There are relatively few studies where increased starch or glucose has been provided through infusion to early lactation dairy cows to determine effects on milk production or body energy balance. However, in early lactation dairy cows incremental infusion of up to 2 kg/d of starch into the duodenum increased milk yield linearly, but decreased milk fat concentration such that there was little effect on milk energy output except for a small increase at the highest level of infusion (Reynolds et al., 2001). This is comparable to the responses to postruminal glucose or ruminal propionate infusion in mid to late lactation cows summarized by Rigout *et al.* (2003). The limited response of milk energy output to starch infusion suggests that the majority of the ME from starch infused was either oxidized or used for body tissue energy deposition, even in early lactation. A similar conclusion was reached in mid-lactation dairy cows infused incrementally with glucose into the jugular vein for 24 days (Al-Trad *et al.*, 2009). As observed for ruminal propionate or postruminal glucose infusion (Rigout *et al.*, 2003), there was an increase in milk yield and protein concentration, but no change in milk energy output and an increase in body weight and condition (Al-Trad *et al.*, 2009). In late lactation cows, infusion of 1.2 kg/d of starch into the abomasum for 14 days had no effect on milk yield or milk energy production, but the ME from the starch infused was used with a very high efficiency (85%) for tissue energy retention, with about 50% of the energy retained as protein (Reynolds *et al.*, 2001). Abomasal starch infusion increased faecal nitrogen concentration and decreased faecal pH, suggesting that a part of the starch infused was resistant to digestion in the small intestine and was fermented in the large intestine, even when a suspension of purified wheat starch was delivered to the abomasum by continuous infusion. In all of these infusion studies, the effects observed are typically expressed relative to a control infusion of water or saline, thus the response is to an increased supply of glucogenic nutrients that provide more ME for metabolism. In contrast, van Knegsel *et al.* (2007a) fed early lactation dairy cows diets of similar NE_l concentration formulated to differ in their supply of lipogenic compared to glucogenic nutrients, primarily by replacing NDF with starch. Measurements of energy metabolism found that cows fed lipogenic diets produced more milk energy and lost more body tissue energy compared to cows fed glucogenic diets, confirming results observed in starch or glucogenic nutrient infusion studies. Similar but smaller differences were observed in a following experiment, but with a smaller contrast in nutrients between lipogenic and glucogenic diets (van Knegsel *et al.*, 2014).

It appears that in lactating dairy cows increased glucogenic nutrient supply through greater starch digestion in the rumen or small intestine is associated with an increase in milk yield and protein concentration, but a reduced milk fat concentration associated with an increase in body tissue energy deposition. This partitioning of dietary ME towards body fat and protein is associated with a change in hormonal status, including increased insulin (Al-Trad *et al.*, 2009; van Knegsel *et al.*, 2007b), associated with less negative body energy balance and improvements in fertility (Garnsworthy *et al.*, 2008). These changes in hormonal status may also contribute to the increase in milk protein concentration observed with greater starch supply, as the response is observed in response to increased propionate or glucose absorption without effects on microbial protein synthesis resulting from increased starch digestion in the rumen. Recent studies have challenged the theory that amino acid use for glucose synthesis in early lactation limits milk protein synthesis (Reynolds *et al.*, 2003; van Vuuren *et al.*, 2014).

To test the theory that a shortage of glucose supply limits milk yield in very early lactation Larsen and Kristensen (2009) initiated abomasal infusions of glucose in the first hours after calving. Increased glucose supply reduced milk yield due to large reductions in DMI that limited the supply of other nutrients and total ME. A reduction in DMI is often observed during intragastric infusions of propionate, glucose or starch in lactating dairy cows (e.g. Rigout *et al.*, 2003). Propionate is an important regulator of DMI through effects on liver oxidative state (Allen *et al.*, 2005), whilst glucose absorbed from the small intestine may affect appetite through direct effects on the hypothalamus, effects on insulin status, or the stimulation of anorexic gut peptides from the small intestinal mucosa (Larsen *et al.*, 2010; Shiriz-Beechey *et al.*, 2014). In this regard increased starch consumption can have negative effects on DMI through increased propionate or glucose absorption, as well as negative effects of reduced ruminal pH on fibre digestion in the rumen (Reynolds *et al.*, 1997; Reynolds, 2006). Depending on the basal diet and amount of starch fed, any effect on total DMI can minimize or negate the potential benefit of increased diet ME concentration for ME intake.

Disadvantages of feeding starch

In addition to being more digestible and having a greater ME concentration, it has long been known that the efficiency of using ME from starch is greater than for ME from forages (Armsby, 1903). However, the rumen has evolved to digest forages, and a risk of feeding starch is the production of excess VFA and in some cases lactate by microbes in the rumen, a reduced milk fat concentration, and associated negative effects of low ruminal pH on rumen function, NDF digestion, DMI, and cow health.

Ruminal acidosis

There has long been concern regarding the potential negative effects of feeding rumen degradable starch, and other NFC substrates, arising from acid accumulation and reduced pH in the rumen. The extent of the pH reduction depends on a number of factors, including rate and extent of ruminal carbohydrate degradation, pattern of intake of diet components (e.g. total mixed rations versus separate concentrate feeding), forage characteristics, and stage of lactation. Clinical ruminal acidosis is a serious condition with major implications for animal welfare and health, but another concern is so-called sub-clinical ruminal acidosis (SARA). A decline in ruminal pH after feeding is normal in ruminants, and especially in lactating dairy cows fed diets containing high proportions of rapidly digestible carbohydrates. However, as VFA are absorbed and buffer is entering the rumen through anion exchange during bicarbonate dependent VFA absorption and through saliva secretion stimulated by postprandial rumination (Dijkstra *et al.*, 2012), the pH of the rumen recovers to 'normal' levels. The definition of SARA is generally recognized as a condition where the amount of time that ruminal pH is below a threshold long enough to be sub-optimal for rumen function. Recent analyses and modelling of available data has suggested that for high yielding dairy cows ruminal pH should have a daily average above 6.2 and ruminal pH below 5.8 for longer than '5.24 h' should be avoided for 'optimal' rumen function (Zebeli *et al.*, 2008). In addition to measurement of ruminal pH, indicators of SARA include decreased milk fat concentration, variable intakes, and abnormal faeces. These are all responses that can be attributed to perturbations of fibre digestion in the rumen. The SARA problem reflects an imbalance between the amount of fermentable substrate in the diet and NDF that is 'effective' at promoting rumination (peNDF), rumen mixing, and saliva production, thus the physical structure of NDF is important. Like SARA, peNDF can be hard to define as the ability of fibre to stimulate rumination and buffer rumen acids is determined by a number of attributes including particle size, shear strength, and specific gravity. The most commonly used method of measuring particle size in dairy cow rations is the Penn State Separator (Heinrichs, 2013), which can be used to measure the distribution of particles in forages and total mixed rations. Zebeli *et al.* (2010) suggested, based on a summarization of ruminal pH data, that to maintain average ruminal pH above 6.2 diets for lactating dairy cows should contain at least 30 to 32% of DM as NDF contained in particles greater than 1.18 mm (peNDF >1.18), with a ratio between peNDF >1.18 and rumen degradable starch content greater than 1.45. In a more recent review, it was suggested that alternatively NDF in larger particles (> 8 mm; peNDF > 8) should be included at no less than 18.5 % of diet DM, but that feeding more than 14.9% of the diet DM as peNDF >8 may reduce DMI (Zebeli *et al.*, 2012) and thus partly negate potential benefits of feeding rumen degradable starch for total energy supply. These contrasting recommendations reflect the challenge of optimizing rumen function by balancing rumen fermentable substrates and peNDF, as the optimal balance for energy intake and milk yield may differ from the optimum for health and milk composition.

In other studies, reduced ruminal fibre digestion with increased diet starch concentration was not related to a reduction in ruminal pH (Pereira and Armentano, 2000; van Vuuren *et al.*, 1999; Table 1). In this regard, an *in vitro* study suggests that the reduction in ruminal fibre digestion is not solely influenced by reduced ruminal pH *per sé*, but is also attributable to increased supply of rumen-available starch (Grant and Mertens, 1992).

Continuous monitoring of ruminal pH shows substantial variability in the postprandial patterns of ruminal pH among cows, with some cows classed as having SARA due to the duration of low ruminal pH, whilst other cows consuming equal amounts of the same diet classed as having normal ruminal pH patterns (Figure 4).

Table 1. Effect of silage quality and supplementing steam-flaked maize (SFM) starch on ruminal pH and ruminal NDF kinetics

Item	Early maturity (394 g NDF/kg DM)		Late maturity (464 g NDF/kg DM)	
	Control	SFM	Control	SFM
Starch intake, kg/d*	0.1	3.6	0.1	3.2
Average ruminal pH⁺	6.2	5.9	6.2	6.2
NDF intake, kg/d*	5.8	5.3	7.0	6.0
NDF Ruminal pool size, kg*	3.7	4.5	4.6	4.8
NDF fractional ruminal degradation rate, /hr*	0.058	0.039	0.053	0.038

*van Vuuren *et al.*, 1999; ⁺unpublished observations.

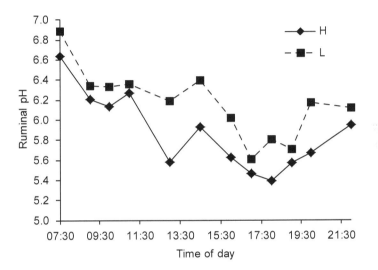

Figure 4. Ruminal pH in high (H) and low (L) yielding dairy cows at similar intakes of the same diet (D. J. Humphries, unpublished observations).

These differences in ruminal pH between cows were associated with differences in ruminal propionate concentration (Figure 5) and may relate to differences in intake pattern, milk yield, VFA absorption, and rate of digesta passage. It appears that some degree of SARA may be 'normal' in early lactation cows with high levels of intake and milk yield that are compensated for by adequate rumination, saliva production, and VFA absorption. However, cows exhibiting variability in their day to day patterns of ruminal pH may be more of a concern. For example, continuous monitoring of ruminal pH using rumen bolus technology in a group of cows fed the same diet in early lactation found that individual cows within the group with higher DMI and milk yield had more regular patterns of ruminal pH decline and recovery from day to day, whilst cows with lower milk yields had more erratic patterns of DMI and

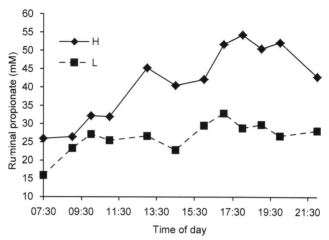

Figure 5. Ruminal propionate concentration in high (H) and low (L) yielding cows at similar intakes of the same diet (D. J. Humphries, unpublished observations).

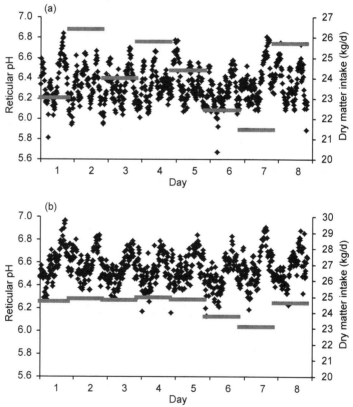

Figure 6. Pattern of reticular pH (black diamonds, primary axis) and dry matter intake (grey bars, secondary axis) measured over an eight-day period for 2 cows: (a) mean pH 6.33, DMI 24.2 kg DM/d, milk yield 36.7 kg/d and (b) mean pH 6.55, DMI 24.4 kg DM/d, milk yield 39.8 kg/d.

pH fluctuation (Figure 6; D. J. Humphries, unpublished observations). It is not known from these anecdotal observations if the differences in patterns between cows simply reflect patterns of intake over time that were affected by other aspects of cow behaviour and physiology during transition, or if the erratic patterns of rumen fermentation contributed to the lower milk yield observed.

In the USA, diet concentrations of NDF and NFC recommended for lactating dairy cows seem low and high, respectively, relative to diets typically fed in Northern Europe. For example, at a forage NDF concentration of 19% of DM recommended total NDF and NFC concentrations are a minimum of 25% NDF and a maximum of 44% NFC (Weiss, 2002). This suggests that recommendations for USA dairy herds may not apply pro rata to conditions in Northern Europe. However, recommendations for the USA are often based on feeding maize grain, which is less degradable than wheat or barley starch and therefore reduces the requirement for peNDF in the ration. It is recommended that when these starch sources are fed or forage particle size is reduced that concentrations of NDF and NFC be adjusted accordingly (Weiss, 2002). In addition, these USA recommendations are based on NFC rather than starch per se, and NFC concentrations of normal rations will be higher than starch concentration. That said, in a survey of high producing commercial dairy herds in the USA starch concentration of the diets fed averaged 27% of DM (Ferraretto *et al.*, 2011). Formulations of rations for dairy cows based on starch concentration and rate and extent of starch digestion require reliable measurements or estimates of starch concentrations, which are difficult to obtain due to the inherent variability of starch analysis (Reynolds *et al.*, 1997).

Feeding food to cows?

Concerns regarding future food security have fuelled discussion regarding the perceived competition between cereal grain use for milk and meat production by animals and human grain consumption, leading some to suggest that in future ruminants should be 'fed no food'. Projections of future global and regional population growth have raised concerns regarding resource availability for food production. Global demand for milk and meat is projected to increase substantially in the next 40 years, along with the demand for cereals for human food consumption and biofuel production (Dijkstra *et al.*, 2013). This has led many to question the ethics of feeding starch to ruminants for milk and meat production in terms of resource use efficiency and associated environmental costs. In reality, much of the cereal grain currently fed to animals is not of milling quality, and supply, demand and cost are and will be a major determinant of amounts of grain fed in rations for dairy cows. In recent years ethanol production has limited maize grain use in US dairy rations where the focus has shifted to feeding more distillers grains and other co-products, thus 'low starch' diets for high-yielding dairy cows have already become a reality for some producers and there is interest in management strategies that maximize starch digestibility, such as feeding exogenous amylase (Weiss *et al.*, 2012; Ferraretto *et al.*, 2011), harvesting grain at lower maturity, processing to increase starch accessibility, or selecting maize varieties with lower virtuousness to increase extent of ruminal digestion (Ferraretto *et al.*, 2013). However, in USA studies evaluating 'reduced starch' versus 'normal starch' diets (Ferraretto *et al.*, 2011) the concentration of starch in the 'reduced starch' treatments was 21%, which is high relative to diets typically fed in many other countries. A great virtue of ruminants is their ability to convert human in-edible, cellulose-based feedstuffs into high quality foods for humans. It is likely that in future economic forces will drive shifts away from cereal grains and towards greater use of co-products from bioenergy production and human food processing in rations for high-yielding dairy cows.

Conclusions

The benefits of feeding starch to high-yielding dairy cows in terms of milk yield and protein concentration have long been recognized and are attributable to greater ME and MP associated with increased digestible energy intake. Benefits of feeding starch include greater total DMI and NE_l supply, but there is a risk that feeding excess NFC relative to peNDF may lead to SARA and associated negative effects on NDF digestion, DMI, milk fat concentration, and health. There is considerable variation in the response of individual animals to variations in diet NDF and NFC concentrations and it appears that some degree of SARA may be 'normal' and well tolerated in higher yielding dairy cows fed highly digestible diets that lead to greater absorption of VFA. Greater glucogenic nutrient supply in early lactation, through increased propionate or glucose absorption, increases milk yield and protein concentration, but reduces milk fat concentration such that the increased ME supplied is used primarily for body energy retention. These positive effects on body energy status are accompanied by changes in hormonal status that have been associated with improved fertility. However, excess body condition in late lactation would be detrimental for the subsequent lactation. In future the amount of grain starch fed to dairy cows will be influenced by requirements for human food and biofuel production and their impact on costs of feeding grains compared to fibrous co-products from human food and biofuel production.

References

Aguerre, M.J., Wattiaux, M.A., Powell, J.M., Broderick, G.A., Arndt, C. (2011) Effect of forage-to-concentrate ratio in dairy cow diets on emission of methane, carbon dioxide, and ammonia, lactation performance, and manure excretion. *Journal of Dairy Science*, **94**, 3081-3093.

Allen, M.A., Bradford, B.J., Harvatine, K.J. (2005) The cow as a model to study intake regulation. *Annual Review of Nutrition*, **25**, 523-547.

Al-Trad, B., Reisberg, K., Wittek, T., Penner, G. B., Alkaassem, A., Gäbel, G., Fürll, M. and Aschenbach, J. R. (2009) Increasing intravenous infusions of glucose improve body condition but not lactation performance in midlactation dairy cows. *Journal of Dairy Science*, **92**, 5645-5658.

Armsby, H.P. (1903) *The Principles of Animal Nutrition*, John Wiley and Sons, New York.

Armsby, HP 1922. *The Nutrition of Farm Animals*, The MacMillan Company, New York.

Armstrong, D.A., Blaxter, K.L., Graham, N.McC. (1960) Fat synthesis from glucose by sheep. *Proceedings of the Nutrition Society*, **19**, xxxi-xxxii.

Bannink, A., Kogut, J., Dijkstra, J., France, J., Kebreab, E., van Vuuren, A.M. and Tamminga, S. (2006) Estimation of the stoichiometry of volatile fatty acid production in the rumen of lactating cows. *Journal of Theoretical Biology*, **238**, 36-51.

Bratzler, J. W. and Forbes, E.B. (1940) The estimation of methane production by cattle. *Journal of Nutrition*, **19**, 611-613.

Butler, W. R. (2000) Nutritional interactions with reproductive performance in dairy cattle. *Animal Reproduction Science*, **60-61**, 449-457

Cassida, K.A., Turner, K.E., Foster, J.G., Hesterman, O.B. (2007) Comparison of detergent fiber methods for forages high in pectin. *Animal Feed Science and Technology*, **135**, 283-295.

Deckardt, K., Khol-Parisini, A. and Zebeli, Q. (2013) Peculiarities of enhancing resistant starch in ruminants using chemical methods: opportunities and challenges. *Nutrients*, **5**, 1970-1988.

Dijkstra J., Reynolds, C.K., Kebreab, E., Bannink, A., Ellis, J.L., France, J. and van Vuuren, A.M. (2013) Challenges in ruminant nutrition: towards minimal nitrogen losses in cattle. In *Energy and protein metabolism and nutrition in sustainable animal production*, pp. 47-58, Edited by J.W. Oltjen, E. Kebreab and H. Lapierre, Wageningen, Academic Publishers, Wageningen, the Netherlands.

Ferraretto, L.F., Crump, P.M. and Shaver, R.D. (2013) Effect of cereal grain type and corn grain harvesting and processing methods on intake, digestion, and milk production by dairy cows through a meta-analysis. *Journal of Dairy Science*, **96**, 533-550.

Ferraretto, L.F., Shaver, R.D, Espineira, M., Gencoglu, H. and Bertics, S.J. (2011) Influence of a reduced-starch diet with or without exogenous amylase on lactation performance by dairy cows. *Journal of Dairy Science*, **94**, 1490-1499.

Firkins, J.L., Eastridge, M.L., St-Pierre, N.R., and Noftsger, S.M. (2001) Effects of grain variability and processing on starch utilization by lactating dairy cattle. *Journal of Animal Science*, **79** (Electronic Supplement), E218-E238.

Garnsworthy, P. C., Sinclair, K.D. and Webb, R. (2008) Integration of physiological mechanisms that influence fertility in dairy cows. *Animal*, **2**, 1144-1152.

Gressley, T.F., Hall, M.B. and Armentano, L.E. (2011) Productivity, digestion, and health responses to hindgut acidosis in ruminants. *Journal of Animal Science*, **89**, 1120-1130.

Grant R.J. and Mertens, D.R. (1992) Influence of buffer pH and raw corn starch addition on in vitro fiber digestion kinetics. *Journal of Dairy Science*, **75**, 2762-2768.

Grummer, R.R. (1993) Etiology of lipid related disorders in periparturient dairy cows. *Journal of Dairy Science,* **76**, 3882-3896.

Heinrichs, J. (2013) The Penn State particle separator. Penn State Extension DSE 2013-186, extension.pse.edu.

Henderson, H.O. and Reaves, P.M. (1954) *Dairy Cattle Feeding and Management.* John Wiley & Sons, New York.

Hindle, V.A., van Vuuren, A.M., Klop, A., Mathijssen-Kamman, A.A., van Gelder, A.H. and Cone, J.W. (2005) Site and extent of starch degradation in the dairy cow – a comparison between in vivo, in situ and in vitro measurements. *Journal of Animal Physiology and Animal Nutrition,* **89**, 158-165.

Hristov, A.N., Oh, J., Firkins, J.L., Dijkstra, J., Kebreab, E., Waghorn, G., Makkar, H.P.S., Adesogan, A.T., Yang, W., Lee, C., Gerber, P.J., Henderson, B. and Tricarico, J.M. (2013) Mitigation of methane and nitrous oxide emissions from animal operations: I. A review of enteric methane mitigation options. *Journal of Animal Science,* **91**, 5045-5069.

Huntington, G. B. (1997) Starch utilization in ruminants. From basics to the bunk. *Journal of Animal Science,* **75**, 852-867.

Ingvartsen, K.L and Andersen, J.B. (2000) Integration of metabolism and intake regulation: A review focusing on periparturient animals. *Journal of Dairy Science,* **83**, 1573-1597.

Knowlton, K.F., Glenn, B.P. and Erdman, R.A. (1998) Performance, ruminal fermentation, and site of starch digestion in early lactation cows fed maize grain harvested and processed differently. *Journal of Dairy Science,* **81**, 1972-1984.

Larsen, M., and Kristensen, N.B. (2009) Effect of abomasal glucose infusion on splanchnic and whole body glucose metabolism in periparturient dairy cows. *Journal of Dairy Science,* **92**, 1071-1083.

Larsen, M., Lund, P., Weisbjerg, M.R. and Hvelplund, T. (2009) Digestion site of starch from cereals and legumes in lactating dairy cows. *Animal Feed Science and Technology,* **153**, 236-248.

Larsen, M., Relling, A. E., Reynolds, C. K., and Kristensen, N. B. (2010) Effect of abomasal glucose infusion on plasma concentrations of gut peptides in periparturient dairy cows. *Journal of Dairy Science,* **93**, 5729-5736.

Li, S., Khafipour, E., Krause, D.O., Kroeker, A., Rodriguez-Lecompte, J.C., Gozho, G.N. and Plaizier, J.C. (2012) Effects of subacute ruminal acidosis challenges on fermentation and endotoxins in the rumen and hindgut of dairy cows. *Journal of Dairy Science,* **95**, 294-303.

Matthé, A., Lebzien, P., Hric, I., Flachowsky, G., and Sommer, A. (2001) Effect of starch application into the proximal duodenum of ruminants on starch digestibility in the small and total intestine. *Archives of Animal Nutrition,* **55**, 351-369.

Mills J.A.N., Kebreab E., Yates C.M., Crompton L.A., Cammell S.B., Dhanoa M.S., Agnew R.E. and France J. (2003) Alternative approaches to predicting methane emissions from dairy cows. *Journal of Animal Science,* **81**, 3141-3150.

Mills, J.A.N., Crompton, L.A., Bannink, A., Tamminga, S., Moorby, J. and Reynolds, C.K. (2009) Predicting methane emissions and nitrogen excretion from cattle. *Journal of Agricultural Science,* **147**, 741.

Moharrery, A., Larsen, M. and Weisbjerg, M.R. (2014) Starch digestion in the rumen, small intestine, and hind gut of dairy cows – A meta-analysis. *Animal Feed Science and Technology*, **192**, 1-14.

Nocek, J.E. and Tamminga, S. (1991) Site of digestion of starch in the gastrointestinal tract of dairy cows and its effect on milk yield and composition. *Journal of Dairy Science*, **74**, 3598-3629.

Oba, M. and Allen, M.S. (2003) Effects of corn grain conservation method on ruminal digestion kinetics for lactating dairy cows at two dietary starch concentrations. *Journal of Dairy Science*, **86**, 184-194.

Owens, F.N., Zinn, R.A. and Kim, Y.K. (1986) Limits to starch digestion in the ruminant small intestine. *Journal of Animal Science,* **63**, 1634–1648.

Pereira, M.N. and L. E. Armentano, L.E. (2000) Partial Replacement of Forage with Nonforage Fiber Sources in Lactating Cow Diets. II. Digestion and Rumen Function. *Journal of Dairy Science*, **83**, 2876–2887.

Phipps, R.H., Sutton, J.D., Humphries, D.J. and Jones, A.K. (2001) A comparison of the effects of cracked wheat and sodium hydroxide treated wheat on food intake, milk production and rumen digestion in dairy cows given maize silage diets. *Animal Science,* **72**, 585–594.

Reynolds, C.K. (2004) Metabolic consequences of increasing milk yield – revisiting Lorna. In *Dairying – Using Science to Meet Consumer's Needs*, pp 73-84 Edited by E. Krebreab, J. Mills, and D. Beever, Nottingham University Press, Nottingham.

Reynolds, C. K. (2006) Production and metabolic effects of site of starch digestion in lactating dairy cattle. *Animal Feed Science and Technology,* **130**, 78-94.

Reynolds, C.K., Cammell, S. B., Humphries, D. J., Beever, D. E., Sutton, J. D. and Newbold, J. R. (2001) Effects of post-rumen starch infusion on milk production and energy metabolism in dairy cows. *Journal of Dairy Science,* **84**, 2250-2259.

Reynolds, C.K., Sutton, J.D. and Beever, D.E. (1997) Effects of feeding starch to dairy cows on nutrient availability and production. In *Recent Advances in Animal Nutrition -1997*, pp 105-134. Edited by P. C. Garnsworthy and J. Wiseman. University of Nottingham Press, Nottingham.

Reynolds, C.K., Aikman, P.C., Lupoli, B., Humphries, D.J. and Beever, D.E. (2003) Splanchnic metabolism of dairy cows during the transition from late gestation through early lactation. *Journal of Dairy Science*, **86**, 1201-1217.

Reynolds, C. K., Crompton, L.A., Mills, J.A.N., Humphries, D.J., Kirton, P., Relling, A.E., Misselbrook, T.H., Chadwick, D.R. and Givens, D.I. (2010) Effects of diet protein level and forage source on energy and nitrogen balance and methane and nitrogen excretion in lactating dairy cows. In *Proceedings of the 3rd International Symposium on Energy and Protein Metabolism*, pp 463-464. Edited by G. M. Corvetto. EAAP Publication Number 127, Wageningen Academic Publishers, The Netherlands.

Rigout, S., Hurtaud, C., Lemosquet, S., Bach, A. and Rulquin, H. (2003) Lactational effect of propionic acid and duodenal glucose in cows. *Journal of Dairy Science,* **86**, 243-253.

Shirazi-Beechey S.P. and D. Bravo. (2014) Nutrient sensing and signalling in the gastrointestinal tract. *British Journal of Nutrition*, **111**, S1-S2.

Theurer, C.B., Huber, J.T., Delgado-Elorduy, A. and Wanderley, R. (1999) Invited review: summary of steam-flaking corn or sorghum grain for lactating dairy cows. *Journal of Dairy Science*, **82**, 1950-1959.

van Knegsel, A. T. M., van den Brand, H., Dijkstra, J., Van Straalen, W.M., Heetkamp, M.J.W., Tamminga, S. and Kemp, B. (2007a) Dietary energy source in dairy cows in early lactation: Energy partitioning and milk composition. *Journal of Dairy Science*, **90**, 1467-1476.

van Knegsel, A. T. M., van den Brand, H., Graat, E.A.M., Dijkstra, J., Jorritsma, R. Decuypere, E., Tamminga, S. and Kemp, B. (2007b) Dietary energy source in dairy cows in early lactation: Metabolites and metabolic hormones. *Journal of Dairy Science*, **90**, 1477-1485.

van Knegsel, A.T.M., Remmelink, G.J., Jorjong, S., Fievez, V. and Kemp, B. (2014) Effect of dry period length and dietary energy source on energy balance, milk yield, and milk composition of dairy cows. *Journal of Dairy Science*, **97**, 1499-1512.

van Vuuren, A. M., Hindle, V.A., Klop, A. and Cone, J.W. (2010) Effect of maize starch concentration in the diet on starch and cell wall digestion in the dairy cow. *Journal of Animal Physiology and Animal Nutrition*, **94**, 319-329.

van Vuuren, A.M., Klop, A., van der Koelen, C.J., and de Visser, H. (1999) Starch and stage of maturity of grass silage: Site of digestion and intestinal nutrient supply in dairy cows. *Journal of Dairy Science*, **82**, 143-152.

van Vuuren, A. M., Dijkstra, J., Reynolds, C.K. and Lemosquet, S. (2014) Nitrogen efficiency and amino acid requirements in dairy cattle. In *Recent Advances in Animal Nutrition - 2014*, pp 49-62. Edited by P. C. Garnsworthy and J. Wiseman. Context Products, Packington, UK.

Waldo, D.R. (1973) Extent and partition of cereal grain starch digestion in ruminants. *Journal of Animal Science*, **37**, 1062-1074.

Washburn, L. E. and S. Brody, S. (1937) Growth and Development. XLII. Methane, hydrogen, and carbon dioxide production in the digestive tract of ruminants in relation to respiratory exchange. Research Bulletin 263. University of Missouri Agricultural Experiment Station.

Weisbjerg, M.R., Bolas, M.V., Huhtala, K., Larsen, M. and Hvelplund, T. (2011) Comparison of in situ and in vitro methods for assessment of in vivo rumen starch degradation. In *Avances in Animal Biosciences Volume 2 Part 2, Proceedings of the 8th International Conference on Nutrition of the Herbivores*, p 325. Cambridge University Press, UK.

Weiss, B. (2002) Protein and carbohydrate utilization by lactating dairy cows. *Proceedings of the Southeast Dairy Herd Management Conference*, pp 72-80.

Weiss, W.P., Steinberg, W. and Engstrom, M.A. (2012) Milk production and nutrient digestibility by dairy cows when fed exogenous amylase with coarsely ground dry corn. *Journal of Dairy Science*, **94**, 2492-2499.

Zebeli, Q., Dijkstra, J., Tafaj, M., Steingass, H., Ametaj, B.N. and Drochner, W. (2008) Modeling the adequacy of dietary fiber in dairy cows based on the responses of ruminal pH and milk fat production to composition of the diet. *Journal of Dairy Science*, **91**, 2046-2066.

Zebeli, Q., Mansmann, D., Steingass, H., and Ametaj, B.N. (2010) Balancing diets for physically effective fibre and ruminally degradable starch: A key to lower the risk of sub-acute rumen acidosis and improve productivity of dairy cattle. *Livestock Science*, **127**, 1-10.

Zebeli, Q., Aschenbach, J.R. Tafaj, M. Boguhn, J., Ametaj, B.N. and Rochner, W. (2012) Role of physically effective fiber and estimation of dietary fiber adequacy in high-producing dairy cattle. *Journal of Dairy Science,* **95**, 1041-1056.

Zom, R.L.G., André, G. and van Vuuren, A.M. (2012) Development of a model for the prediction of feed intake by dairy cows: 1. Prediction of feed intake. *Livestock Science,* **143**, 43-57.

4

Nitrogen Efficiency and Amino Acid Requirements in Dairy Cattle

A. M. VAN VUUREN*, J. DIJKSTRA[†], C. K. REYNOLDS[‡] AND
S. LEMOSQUET[§]

*Wageningen UR Livestock Research, Wageningen, the Netherlands; [†]Animal
Nutrition Group, Wageningen University, the Netherlands; [‡]University of Reading,
School of Agriculture, Policy and Development, Earley Gate, Reading, RG6 6AR,
UK; [§] INRA UMR1348 Pegase, 35590 Saint-Gilles, France

Introduction

For more than 40 years, protein nutrition and metabolism in livestock animals has been a major subject for research. The beneficial effect of dietary protein on livestock performance and the relatively high value of protein-rich ingredients were main reasons to assess the optimum dietary protein level. Scientists have long been aware of the high manure nitrogen (N) excretion and relatively low N use efficiency of livestock and the impact of manure N on the environment. In more recent years, public concerns over the impact of land use changes for feed protein production in combination with predicted increase in the demand for animal protein have become another stimulus to assess the optimum dietary protein level balancing animal performance and the ecological footprint of livestock production.

Although ruminants are less efficient in feed protein use than monogastric livestock, the human edible protein efficiency is substantially higher than for monogastrics and is usually greater than 1.0, indicating that ruminants add to the total human food supply (Dijkstra et al., 2013b). This protein gain by ruminants results from the nature of plant proteins consumed by ruminants. Plant proteins for ruminants are often embedded in high-fibre forages (e.g. grass, clover) and high-fibre, inedible residues of the food industry (e.g. expellers, brewer's grains, gluten feeds) that are not potential foods for humans.

However, competition for arable land between crop and forage production may affect the overall sustainability of cattle operations. Although high-producing dairy cattle have a relatively high protein use efficiency by diluting maintenance requirements over more milk (Dijkstra et al., 2013b), the required production of highly-digestible home-grown forages to enable high levels of milk production typically requires high levels of N fertilizer which has a negative environmental impact at farm level, or requires protein meal supplementation. Therefore, the complete farm N cycle including feed, manure, soil and, as the principal component, the dairy cow should be taken into account when discussing protein use efficiency of dairy production systems.

This chapter will focus on new developments and perspectives of protein and amino acid (AA) metabolism in the dairy cow that affect N efficiency, including ruminal microbial protein synthesis, efficiency at which absorbed AA are utilised in intermediary metabolism, and AA requirements for milk protein synthesis and other processes.

N intake, utilisation, excretion and environmental impacts (NH_3, NO_2, N_2O)

In various studies a positive relationship between N intake or diet N concentration (Figure 1) and milk N secretion has been reported (Kebreab *et al.*, 2001; Huhtanen and Hristov, 2009; Kebreab *et al.*, 2010). This relationship apparently suggests that with increasing N intake milk protein secretion increases. However, it should be recognised that these desktop studies were based on data from experiments in which feeds were formulated according to the milk production level of the cows used in these studies, often using protein sources with varying level of degradability within individual experiments. Thus, the reported relationships between N intake or diet N concentration and milk protein secretion are mainly influenced by the research treatments employed. Indeed, in their meta-analysis, Huhtanen and Hristov (2009) reported that only in 7 of the 31 experiments studying the effect of dietary crude protein (CP) concentration, was CP concentration significantly and positively related to milk protein secretion. In 5 of those 7 studies, the effect of diet CP concentration on milk yield was attributable to an increase in diet dry matter (DM) intake. According to NRC (2001), milk yield increases quadratically with increased dietary CP concentration, with maximum milk production obtained at 230 g CP/kg diet DM. Dietary CP concentration was only weakly correlated with milk protein yield though and maximal at 220 g CP/kg diet DM.

Both Huhtanen and Hristov (2009) and Kebreab *et al.* (2010) reported a relatively low efficiency by which extra feed N (metabolisable protein [MP] or CP) is secreted in milk. Huhtanen and Hristov (2009) reported that on average 25% of feed protein was secreted in milk protein in a North American dataset and 28% in a North European dataset; in studies at the University of Reading a recovery of diet CP as milk protein of only 20% was observed (Kebreab *et al.*, 2010). These relatively low efficiencies can be an indication for over-supply of dietary CP in many of these experiments, but may also be due to low marginal efficiencies by which MP is incorporated into

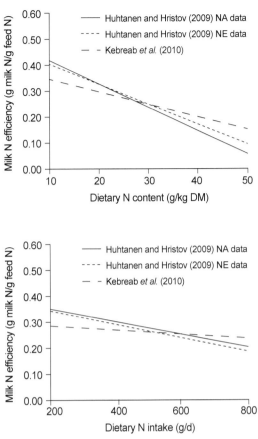

Figure 1. Effect of dietary N content and dietary N intake on milk N efficiency based on equations derived by Huhtanen and Hristov (2009) (NA, North America; NE, North Europe) and by Kebreab *et al.* (2010)

milk protein, being 38% or lower in these experiments. These marginal efficiencies are much lower than the overall MP use efficiency for milk production assumed in various protein evaluation systems (64 to 68%) and also much lower than theoretical maximum efficiency (85%) (see Dijkstra *et al.*, 2013c).

Various authors studied the relationship between N intake and N excretion in faeces and urine. Because urinary N excretion has a higher impact on environmental pollution than faecal N excretion, only the relationship between N intake and urinary N will be presented briefly. In the analyses of data, urinary N excretion increases linearly or exponentially with increasing N intake. From these equations it can be calculated that at a DM intake of 24 kg/d with 170 g CP/kg DM, (~ 640 g of N/d), 40 to 50% of ingested N will be excreted in urine. Within the 27 member states of the European Union, annually more than 150 million tonnes of milk are produced.

Assuming a milk protein content of 33 g/kg and a milk protein efficiency of 25% it can be calculated that dairy cows within the EU27 excrete per year, 1.2 to 1.5 x 10^9 kg of urinary N! Volatilisation as NH_3 may vary between 3 and 15% of urinary N and as N_2O between < 1 and > 10% (Dijkstra *et al.*, 2013b). Assuming 5% of urinary N is lost as NH_3 then NH_3 loss would be 60 to 75 million kg of N, while a 1.3% loss of urinary N as N_2O would be more than 16 million kg of N per annum within the EU27. Improving overall milk protein efficiency from 25 to 30% would result in a more than 16% reduction in these emissions.

Because supplementing additional protein has only a marginal effect on milk protein yield, but a significant effect on urinary N excretion and hence emissions of NH_3 and N_2O, the question has arisen as how to define the optimal protein level for dairy cattle. This was recognised more than 4 decades ago resulting in the development of new protein evaluation systems that were based on the digestive processes, predicting supply of absorbable protein and minimising N losses in the rumen (Vérité and Peyraud, 1989; Thomas, 2004; van Duinkerken *et al.*, 2011; Volden, 2011). These new protein evaluation systems may in principal enable nutritionists to use smaller safety margins in feed formulation, which would allow a reduction in dietary N levels.

Another development reducing dietary N levels for dairy cows has been a reduction in N fertilizer use, which has resulted in lower CP levels of home-grown forages. However, the reduction in N fertilizer was sometimes accompanied by introduction of legumes for N fixation to compensate for the reduction in DM yield resulting from lower N fertilizer rates, which counteracted effects of the reduction in applied fertilizer N on forage CP concentrations. It is likely that withdrawal of milk quotas within the EU may increase demand for home-grown forages, resulting (within limits set by governments) in a rise in fertilizer N or N-fixing legumes, thereby increasing N losses into the environment as NH_3 and N_2O.

From their analysis to identify maximal possible N efficiency, Dijkstra *et al.* (2013c) concluded that strategies to reduce N losses and improve N efficiency should focus on an optimal supply of rumen degradable N (RDN) and optimal efficiency of utilization of absorbed AA for milk protein synthesis, and these are discussed next.

Inefficiency of microbial protein synthesis

Although the ability of ruminants to convert protein from biomass inedible by humans into edible milk and meat results in positive edible protein efficiency, the conversion via microbial protein synthesis comes at a price. The ruminal microbial population not only converts dietary protein and non-protein-N into digestible microbial protein, but also into other nitrogenous components, such as nucleic acids. Assuming that 25% of microbial CP is present as nucleic acids, it was estimated that conversion of dietary CP into microbial CP results in more than 70 g of inevitable urinary N loss/d by a 650-kg dairy cow, producing 1.3 kg of milk protein/d, with a further 13 g of faecal N loss/d in undigested nucleic acid N (Dijkstra *et al.*, 2013c). Moreover, the levels of ammonia-N, AA-N or peptide-N in the rumen required for maximal microbial protein synthesis give rise to a net unavoidable N loss in urine of 35 g/d. Such inevitable losses depend on various factors, including feed intake level, and abating these losses requires protein evaluation systems to represent the dynamics of microbial protein synthesis in a proper way. Unfortunately, current protein evaluation systems have only limited value in providing guidance to reduce these losses of N arising from rumen microbial metabolism. To improve upon current prediction schemes, new feeding systems need to be based on mechanisms that govern the response of animals to nutrients, by quantitatively describing metabolite supply at a more detailed level than the current aggregated components.

One source of non-protein N for ruminal microorganisms is urea that has been recycled from blood into the rumen. Urea recycling is via saliva and via the rumen wall. Between 30 and almost 100% of all urea-N entering the blood pool is returned to the gut (Reynolds and Kristensen, 2008). Even when 100% of urea is returned to the gut, urinary N excretion still occurs, but the N is then excreted primarily in forms other than urea, including purine derivatives, hippuric acid, creatine and creatinine (Dijkstra *et al.*, 2013b). Dijkstra *et al.*, (2013a) compared four models to predict urea-N recycling. In 3 of the 4 models, dietary CP level had no effect on the total amount of urea-N recycled into the rumen (Dijkstra *et al.*, 2013a). In an experimental study with dairy cows, blood urea-N concentration did not affect the amount of urea-N recycled, indicating an effect of blood N concentration – and consequently dietary CP level – on the extraction rate of blood urea-N by the rumen, but not on the total amount of N recycled to the rumen (Røjen *et al.*, 2011). Thus, dairy cattle appear unable to up-regulate urea-N transport sufficiently to fully compensate for reduced RDN content of the diet and maintain milk protein yield.

Synchronising the availability of energy (carbohydrates) and nitrogenous compounds (ammonia, AA) has been advocated as a means to improve microbial protein synthesis based on positive effects in sheep (Sinclair *et al.*, 1993). Under practical conditions, however, a response to synchronised diets has not been observed (Hall and Huntington, 2008). The recycling of urea-N buffers effects of asynchronous energy and N supply to the rumen, which may explain the general lack of positive response to attempts to synchronize rumen energy and N supply reported in the literature. In contrast, imposing asynchrony through infrequent supplementation or oscillating dietary protein concentration, has not negatively affected production responses unless the frequency of supplementation is less than once every 3 d (Reynolds and Kristensen, 2008). Synchronising the availability of energy and RDN may be important for rapidly degradable substrates, but an extra need for more slowly degradable CP can be disputed, because the relatively slow growth rate of cell wall degrading micro-organisms will require only small amounts of available N, which can be met by the reflux of urea-N (van Vuuren and Tamminga, 2001). Nowadays, high-yielding cows are mainly fed *ad libitum*. Cows fed *ad libitum* will consume their ration in frequent meals resulting in a regular supply of available substrates. If concentrates are fed by computerized concentrate feeders, both partial mixed ration and concentrates should be well balanced in available energy and RDP.

Inefficiency of utilisation of absorbed AA

During the last 3 to 4 decades protein evaluation systems have been modified extensively, resulting in complex calculations to predict the supplies of protein or AA that are absorbed and/or available to the mammary gland based on dietary composition. Much less attention has been given to estimating optimum AA requirements and their relationship with supply of other nutrients. Absorbed AA will be used for maintenance (e.g. turnover of cells, cell organelles and enzymes), for protein retention (gestation, growth) and for milk protein synthesis. Surplus AA will be deaminated and oxidised yielding energy, glucose and other metabolites. Because AA can be used for hepatic gluconeogenesis, it has been postulated that due to the rapidly increased glucose requirement postpartum, supply of available AA to the mammary gland may be limited during the period of a so-called negative energy balance. However, such a mechanism appears disputable, since it is more likely that the postpartum cow prioritises secretion of nutrients for her offspring. Indeed the contribution of AA to gluconeogenesis in the first week postpartum was relatively small, accounting on average for 2.5% of total hepatic glucose release by essential AA (EAA) and 14% by non-essential AA (nEAA) (Larsen and Kristensen, 2013). In addition, Reynolds *et al.* (2003) found no evidence of a requirement for a greater contribution of AA to hepatic glucose release in early lactation, apart from a greater measured contribution of alanine (Table 1). Besides, after a decline in plasma AA concentrations during the first week postpartum, blood concentrations of most EAA and nEAA recovered within 3 weeks, except for glutamine, methionine and phenylalanine (Meijer *et al.*, 1995).

It has now been accepted that liver and intestinal tissues are reactive users of AA that have not been incorporated in milk or body proteins and not active regulators of AA availability to the mammary gland (see (Calsamiglia *et al.*, 2010). Indeed, in mid-lactation dairy cows, excess of AA increased whole body glucose entry rate (Lemosquet *et al.*, 2009a; Lemosquet *et al.*, 2009b; Galindo *et al.*, 2011), suggesting that gluconeogenesis can utilise surplus AA, but mammary glucose uptake was not increased in those studies. Similar studies have shown that increased provision of AA to lactating dairy cows via abomasal infusion cows reduces liver lactate removal,

Table 1. Maximal net contributions of glucose precursors (excluding amino acids other than alanine) removed to glucose released (% of total) by the liver of transition dairy cows (Reynolds *et al.*, 2003)

Item	Average day relative to calving						SEM
	-19	-9	11	21	33	83	
Propionate	55.2	43.5	55.8	49.0	57.6	66.4	7.0
Lactate	18.5	22.7	21.1	16.9	15.6	8.0	2.7
Alanine	3.1	2.3	5.5	3.0	1.5	1.7	0.6
Glycerol	2.3	3.0	3.6	2.4	1.5	0.4	0.7
Triglyceride glycerol	-0.2	1.5	0.2	0.0	0.1	-0.1	0.5
i-Butyrate	1.7	1.4	1.3	1.1	1.4	1.6	0.5
n-Valerate	2.8	2.4	3.3	2.3	2.8	3.0	0.6
Total	83.4	76.8	88.9	74.7	80.5	81.8	7.5

suggesting reduced Cori cycling of glucose and lactate between peripheral tissues and the liver (Reynolds, 2002).

Thus, the question remains how uptake of AA by the mammary gland can be optimized to avoid an undesirable surplus of AA and minimize excretion of urinary N. Various reasons for suboptimal AA uptake by the mammary gland have been postulated, such as a suboptimal profile of AA supplied to the mammary gland; suboptimal synchronisation of available energy and AA for the mammary gland and asynchrony between available nutrients; and the activity of anabolic pathways in mammary cells (Arriola Apelo *et al.*, 2014a), resulting in suboptimal uptake or cellular utilisation of AA.

Amino acid profile

A shortage of one or more EAA in relation to the other EAA and their requirements has been postulated for many years as a limit for mammary protein synthesis and appears the main driver for including rumen-protected AA considered as first-limiting, especially when reducing dietary CP content (e.g. Broderick *et al.*, 2009). This theory is often presented as a barrel made of staves with different lengths, which represent supply of an AA relative to the ideal profile (see Cant *et al.*, 2003), where the ideal AA profile refers to the AA profile of milk protein. Methionine and lysine are considered to be the first limiting AA for milk production and a large number of studies on the effect of supplementing these AA, protected from rumen fermentation, have been reported. A recent meta-analysis of effects of rumen-protected methionine (RPM) included 36 studies (Patton, 2010). Adding RPM to rations of dairy cows overall resulted in an increase in true milk protein content of 0.7 g/kg of milk and an increase in true milk protein yield of 27 g/d. These and other responses to RPM were not influenced by supply of lysine or by other dietary factors (levels of NDF and CP, and energy balance); but of considerable interest is the observation that these responses did not depend on amount of RPM fed or on calculated severity of methionine deficiency. Fewer studies have been performed with lysine, and responses to supplementing rumen-protected lysine have been variable, attributed to the influence of other dietary characteristics (Mullins *et al.*, 2013; Paz *et al.*, 2013) or stage of lactation, possibly changing the priority in AA partitioning (Robinson *et al.*, 2011). In some studies, histidine has been considered as the first-limiting AA (Vanhatalo *et al.*, 1999). A relative low duodenal supply of histidine may result when dairy cows rely mainly on microbial protein, which is relatively low in histidine (Boisen *et al.*, 2000). Such conditions are favoured when feeding diets high in RDP, such as relatively wet grass silages.

A mixture of methionine, lysine, histidine and leucine, infused duodenally, increased milk protein output in dairy cattle (with a milk yield of approximately 30 kg/d) by 0.07 kg/d (Haque *et al.*, 2012). In this experiment the response to infusion of these 4 EAA was not dependent on the basic MP level of the diet (48.6 versus 58.4 g PDI/Mcal NEL), nor on additional duodenal infusion of isoleucine, valine, phenylalanine, tryptophan and tyrosine. The positive response to EAA infusion at the higher MP level suggests that supplying these EAA has a more specific effect than simply compensating for a possible deficiency in certain EAA. It should be noticed that some EAA (lysine, isoleucine, leucine, valine and arginine) are metabolised within the mammary gland contributing to nEAA syntheses and providing energy (Mepham, 1982). Their contribution to mammary metabolism varies, as shown by the increase in their uptake to output ratio when increasing MP supplies (Lapierre *et al.*, 2012). In addition, competitive inhibition of uptake of AA by the same transporters in the mammary gland may result in decreased milk protein synthesis rate and in this respect again supplying the correct profile of AA to the mammary gland is of large importance (Maas *et al.*, 1998). This also suggests that supplying optimum amounts of EAA to the mammary gland may be more complicated than simply providing amounts equivalent to their secretion in milk protein.

Synchrony between energy and AA supply at mammary gland level

A shortage of ATP yielding nutrients is another possible reason for inefficient utilisation of AA by the mammary gland. In the meta-analysis of Kebreab *et al.* (2010), metabolisable energy (ME) intake as a covariate with N intake had a significant positive effect on milk N efficiency and a negative effect on urinary N excretion, but ME had no significant effect on predicted faecal N excretion. Kebreab et al. (2010) suggested that the extra energy stimulated microbial protein synthesis, but since there was no effect of ME intake as a covariate on faecal N excretion, a positive effect of additional absorbed energy at intermediary metabolism level cannot be excluded.

The relationship between energy and AA supply (MP) has been incorporated into the INRA protein evaluation system (INRA, 2007) to limit urinary N excretion.

This relationship is based on experiments which showed that above the threshold of 100-105 g of PDIE (Intestinal Digestible Protein) per 1.7 Mcal of NE_L, the ratio between urinary N and milk N increases exponentially (Vérité and Delaby, 2000).

Experiments have been performed to study the effect of glucose and acetate infusions on efficiency of AA secretion in milk protein. Post-ruminal glucose infusion resulted in contradictory responses, varying from positive to negative, with no clear explanation, as has been discussed recently (Safayi and Nielsen, 2013). Dietary starch supplementation may increase milk protein yield (Higgs *et al.*, 2013), but it can be disputed whether this effect is due to higher microbial protein synthesis in the rumen or higher energy supply to the mammary gland. On the other hand, postruminal starch infusion was associated with an increase in body tissue energy and N deposition in lactating dairy cows, but not with greater milk protein production (Reynolds *et al.*, 2001). Infusion of acetate in lactating dairy goats did compensate for insufficient EAA supply in early-lactation, but not in late-lactation (Safayi and Nielsen, 2013). Ruminal infusion of propionate in lactating dairy cows decreased leucine oxidation when AA supply was given in excess by duodenal infusion of casein (Raggio *et al.*, 2006). Overall, effects of energetic nutrients are difficult to understand, perhaps because the mammary gland presents a high metabolic flexibility to utilize all types of nutrients (including AA) as energy sources (Lobley, 2007).

Activity of metabolic pathways in mammary gland

Protein synthesis is regulated by many mechanisms and pathways related to amongst others AA transport into the epithelial cells, activation through phosphorylation, transcription of DNA and RNA, and elongation, with the mammalian target of rapamycin (mTOR) pathway in a central role. Nutrients may influence these processes at different levels, either directly or indirectly. As an example, glucose infusion may affect AA synthesis either directly by influencing the mTOR pathway or indirectly through an effect of insulin on phosphorylation processes (Arriola Apelo *et al.*, 2014a).

In recent studies, the specific effect of other nutrients, besides glucose, on the mTOR pathway has been demonstrated. Amongst the EAA, leucine and isoleucine were identified as regulatory nutrients of the mTOR pathway, but the protein signalling response to isoleucine and leucine were conditioned by antagonisms between these and with other AA (Arriola Apelo *et al.*, 2014b). In vitro studies showed that total mTOR protein expression is increased by addition of lysine alone and in combination with methionine, with the highest casein production at a methionine:lysine ratio of 1:3 (Nan *et al.*, 2014), remarkably close to the required methionine:lysine ratio for MP in protein evaluation systems.

Specific amino acid use

Besides building blocks for proteins, EAA may also be functional nutrients. As an example, methionine can also be activated in sulphur-adenosylmethionine, a methyl donor for transmethylation reactions, implying an interaction between methionine, choline, folic acid and betaine (Bertolo and McBreairty, 2013). Thus, improving methionine supply could have a sparing effect on choline (and vice versa) and consequently improve hepatic fat metabolism and animal performance in early lactation (Zom *et al.*, 2011; Goselink *et al.*, 2013).

Conclusion

To reduce the environmental impact of N excretion by dairy cattle, optimising N intake should be the main nutritional strategy. Although new protein evaluation systems enable a reduction in safety margins, these systems are not yet fully exploited. The concept that converting a MP system into a metabolisable AA system would enable a further reduction in dietary N seems acceptable, but our knowledge of variation in microbial protein AA composition and in composition of AA available for milk syntheses, and of the role of AA and other nutrients in regulating pathways for protein synthesis in the mammary gland, is still too limited for development of such a metabolisable AA system. Supplementing individual (rumen-protected) AA based on the "barrel concept" appears to be scientifically less clear. Positive effects of supplemental AA may be attributed to specific functions of these AA resulting in activation of the protein synthetic pathways.

References

Arriola Apelo S.I., Knapp J.R. and Haningan M.D. (2014a) Current representation and future trends of predicting amino acid utilization in the lactating dairy cow. *Journal of Dairy Science* **97**, 18.

Arriola Apelo S.I., Singer L.M., Lin X.Y., McGilliard M.L., St-Pierre N.R. and Hanigan M.D. (2014b) Isoleucine, leucine, methionine, and threonine effects on mammalian target of rapamycin signaling in mammary tissue. *Journal of Dairy Science* **97**, 1047-1056.

Bertolo R.F. and McBreairty L.E. (2013) The nutritional burden of methylation reactions. *Current Opinion in Clinical Nutrition and Metabolic Care* **16**, 102-108.

Boisen S., Hvelplund T. and Weisbjerg M.R. (2000) Ideal amino acid profiles as a basis for feed protein evaluation. *Livestock Production Science* **64**, 239-251.

Broderick G.A., Stevenson M.J. and Patton R.A. (2009) Effect of dietary protein concentration and degradability on response to rumen-protected methionine in lactating dairy cows. *Journal of Dairy Science* **92**, 2719-2728.

Calsamiglia S., Ferret A., Reynolds C.K., Kristensen N.B. and van Vuuren A.M. (2010) Strategies for optimizing nitrogen use by ruminants. *Animal* **4**, 1184-1196.

Cant J.R., Berthiaume R., Lapierre H., Luimes P.H., McBride B.W. and Pacheco D. (2003) Responses of the bovine mammary glands to absorptive supply of single amino acids. *Canadian Journal of Animal Science* **83**, 341-355.

Dijkstra J., Bannink A., France J. and Ellis J.L. (2013a) Improved prediction of recycling of urea into the rumen of cattle. In *Report EU project Reducing Nitrogen Excretion Dairy Cattle*, available from: http://www.rednex-fp7.eu/Docs/Deliverable%20Reports/D%205.5.pdf.

Dijkstra J., Oenema O., van Groenigen J.W., Spek J.W., van Vuuren A.M. and Bannink A. (2013b) Diet effects on urine composition of cattle and N_2O emissions. *Animal* **7** Suppl 2, 292-302.

Dijkstra J., Reynolds C.K., Kebreab E., Bannink A., Ellis J.L., France J. and van Vuuren A.M. (2013c) Challenges in ruminant nutrition: towards minimal nitrogen losses in cattle. In *Energy and protein metabolism and nutrition in sustainable animal production* (eds. J.W. Oltjen, E. Kebreab and H. Lapierre), pp. 47-58, Wageningen Academic Publishers, Wageningen, the Netherlands.

Galindo C.E., Ouellett D.R., Pellerin D., Lemosquet S., Ortigues-Marty I. and Lapierre H. (2011) Effect of amino acid or casein supply on whole-body, splanchnic, and mammary glucose kinetics in lactating dairy cows. *Journal of Dairy Science* **94**, 5558-5568.

Goselink R.M.A., van Baal J., Widjaja H.C.A., Dekker R.A., Zom R.L.G., de Veth M.J. and van Vuuren A.M. (2013) Effect of rumen-protected choline supplementation on liver and adipose gene expression during the transition period in dairy cattle. *Journal of Dairy Science* **96**, 1102-1116.

Hall M.B. and Huntington G.B. (2008) Nutrient synchrony: Sound in theory, elusive in practice. *Journal of Animal Science* **86** E287-292.

Haque M.N., Rulquin H., Andrade A., Faverdin P., Peyraud J.L. and Lemosquet S. (2012) Milk protein synthesis in response to the provision of an "ideal" amino acid profile at 2 levels of metabolizable protein supply in dairy cows. *Journal of Dairy Science* **95**, 5876-5887.

Higgs R.J., Sheahan A.J., Mandok K., Van Amburgh M.E. and Roche J.R. (2013) The effect of starch-, fiber-, or sugar-based supplements on nitrogen utilization in grazing dairy cows. *Journal of Dairy Science* **96**, 3857-3866.

Huhtanen P. and Hristov A.N. (2009) A meta-analysis of the effects of dietary protein concentration and degradability on milk protein yield and milk N efficiency in dairy cows. *Journal of Dairy Science* **92**, 3222-3232.

INRA (2007) *Nutrition of Cattle, Sheep and Goats: Animal Needs–Values of Feeds*. Quae Editions, Paris, France.

Kebreab E., France J., Beever D.E. and Castillo A.R. (2001) Nitrogen pollution by dairy cows and its mitigation by dietary manipulation. *Nutrient Cycling in Agroecosystems* **60**, 275-285.

Kebreab E., Strathe A.B., Dijkstra J., Mills J.A.N., Reynolds C.K., Crompton L.A., Yan T. and France J. (2010) Energy and protein interactions and their effect on nitrogen excretion in dairy cows. In *3rd EAAP International Symposium on Energy and Protein Metabolism and Nutrition*, pp. 417-425

Lapierre H., Lobley G.E., Doepel L., Raggio G., Rulquin H. and Lemosquet S. (2012) Triennial Lactation Symposium: Mammary metabolism of amino acids in dairy cows. Journal of *Animal Science* **90**, 1708-1721.

Larsen M. and Kristensen N.B. (2013) Precursors for liver gluconeogenesis in periparturient dairy cows. *Animal* **7**, 1640-1650.

Lemosquet S., Delamaire E., Lapierre H., Blum J.W. and Peyraud J.L. (2009a) Effects of glucose, propionic acid, and nonessential amino acids on glucose metabolism and milk yield in Holstein dairy cows. *Journal of Dairy Science* **92**, 3244-3257.

Lemosquet S., Raggio G., Lobley G.E., Rulquin H., Guinard-Flament J. and Lapierre H. (2009b) Whole-body glucose metabolism and mammary energetic nutrient metabolism in lactating dairy cows receiving digestive infusions of casein and propionic acid. *Journal of Dairy Science* **92**, 6068-6082.

Lobley G.E. (2007) Protein-energy interaction: horizontal aspects. In *Energy and Protein Metabolism and Nutrition*, Wageningen, The Netherlands, pp. 445-461.

Maas J.A., France J., Dijkstra J., Bannink A. and McBride B.W. (1998) Application of a mechanistic model to study competitive inhibition of amino acid uptake by the lactating bovine mammary gland. *Journal of Dairy Science* **81**, 1724-1734.

Meijer G.A.L., van der Meulen J., Bakker J.G.M., van der Koelen C.J. and van Vuuren A.M. (1995) Free amino-acids in plasma and muscle of high-yielding dairy-cows in early lactation. *Journal of Dairy Science* **78**, 1131-1141.

Mullins C.R., Weber D., Block E., Smith J.F., Brouk M.J. and Bradford B.J. (2013) Supplementing lysine and methionine in a lactation diet containing a high concentration of wet corn gluten feed did not alter milk protein yield. *Journal of Dairy Science* **96**, 5300-5305.

Nan X.M., Bu D.P., Li X.Y., Wang J.Q., Wei H.Y., Hu H., Zhou L.Y. and Loor J.J. (2014) Ratio of lysine to methionine alters expression of genes involved in milk protein transcription and translation and mTOR phosphorylation in bovine mammary cells. *Physiological Genomics* **46**, 268-275.

Patton R.A. (2010) Effect of rumen-protected methionine on feed intake, milk production, true milk protein concentration, and true milk protein yield, and the factors that influence these effects: A meta-analysis. *Journal of Dairy Science* **93**, 2105-2118.

Paz H.A., de Veth M.J., Ordway R.S. and Kononoff P.J. (2013) Evaluation of rumen-protected lysine supplementation to lactating dairy cows consuming increasing amounts of distillers dried grains with solubles. *Journal of Dairy Science* **96**, 7210-7222.

Raggio G., Lobley G.E., Lemosquet S., Rulquin H. and Lapierre H. (2006) Effect of casein and propionate supply on whole body protein metabolism in lactating dairy cows. *Canadian Journal of Animal Science* **86**, 81-89.

Reynolds C.K. (2002) Economics of visceral nutrient metabolism in ruminants – toll keeping or internal revenue service? *Journal of Animal Science* **80**, E74-84.

Reynolds C.K. and Kristensen N.B. (2008) Nitrogen recycling through the gut and the nitrogen economy of ruminants: An asynchronous symbiosis. *Journal of Animal Science* **86**, E293-305.

Reynolds C.K., Aikman P.C., Lupoli B., Humphries D.J. and Beever D.E. (2003) Splanchnic metabolism of dairy cows during the transition from late gestation through early lactation. *Journal of Dairy Science* **86**, 1201-1217.

Reynolds C.K., Cammell S.B., Humphries D.J., Beever D.E., Sutton J.D. and Newbold J.R. (2001) Effects of postrumen starch infusion on milk production and energy metabolism in dairy cows. *Journal of Dairy Science* **84**, 2250-2259.

Robinson P.H., Swanepoel N., Shinzato I. and Juchem S.O. (2011) Productive responses of lactating dairy cattle to supplementing high levels of ruminally protected lysine using a rumen protection technology. *Animal Feed Science and Technology* **168**, 30-41.

Røjen B.A., Theil P.K. and Kristensen N.B. (2011) Effects of nitrogen supply on inter-organ fluxes of urea-N and renal urea-N kinetics in lactating Holstein cows. *Journal of Dairy Science* **94**, 2532-2544.

Safayi S. and Nielsen M.O. (2013) Intravenous supplementation of acetate, glucose or essential amino acids to an energy and protein deficient diet in lactating dairy goats: Effects on milk production and mammary nutrient extraction. *Small Ruminant Research* **112**, 162-173.

Sinclair L.A., Garnsworthy P.C., Newbold J.R. and Buttery P.J. (1993) Effect of synchronizing the rate of dietary energy and nitrogen release on rumen fermentation and microbial protein-synthesis in sheep. *Journal of Agricultural Science* **120**, 251-263.

Thomas C. (2004) *Feed Into Milk—A New Applied Feeding System for Dairy Cows*. Nottingham University Press, Nottingham, UK.

van Duinkerken G., Blok M.C., Bannink A., Cone J.W., Dijkstra J., van Vuuren A.M. and Tamminga S. (2011) Update of the Dutch protein evaluation system for ruminants: the DVE/OEB2010 system. *Journal of Agricultural Science* **149**, 351-367.

van Vuuren A.M. and Tamminga S. (2001) De fysiologische basis voor de minimale onbestendige eiwitbalans in melkveerantsoenen. [Physiological base for the minimal rumen degradable protein balance]. In *CVB-documentatierapport nr 28*, p. 22. Centraal Veevoederbureau, Lelystad, The Netherlands.

Vanhatalo A., Huhtanen P., Toivonen V. and Varvikko T. (1999) Response of dairy cows fed grass silage diets to abomasal infusions of histidine alone or in combinations with methionine and lysine. *Journal of Dairy Science* **82**, 2674-2685.

Vérité R. and Peyraud J-L. (1989) Protein: the PDI systems. In *Ruminant Nutrition: Recommended Allowances and Feed Tables* (ed. R Jarrige), pp. 33-48, INRA/John Libbey Eurotext, London-Paris.

Vérité R. and Delaby L. (2000) Relation between nutrition, performances and nitrogen excretion in dairy cows. *Annales De Zootechnie* **49**, 217-230.

Volden H. (2011) *NorFor - The Nordic Feed Evaluation System*. Wageningen Academic Publishers, Wageningen, The Netherlands.

Zom R.L.G., van Baal J., Goselink R.M.A., Bakker J.A., de Veth M.J. and van Vuuren A.M. (2011) Effect of rumen-protected choline on performance, blood metabolites, and hepatic triacylglycerols of periparturient dairy cattle. *Journal of Dairy Science* **94**, 4016-4027.

5

Manipulating Rumen Fermentation to Improve Efficiency and Reduce Environmental Impact

C JAMIE NEWBOLD, GABRIEL DE LA FUENTE, ALEJANDRO BELANCHE, KENTON HART, ERIC PINLOCHE, TOBY WILKINSON, ELI R SAETNAN AND EVA RAMOS-MORALES

Institute of Biological Environmental and Rural Sciences, Aberystwyth University, Aberystwyth, Ceredigion, SY23 3DD. United Kingdom

Introduction

Microbial fermentation in the rumen plays a central role in the ability of ruminants to utilize fibrous substrates; however rumen fermentation also has potential deleterious environmental consequences as it ultimately leads to the emission of greenhouse gases and breakdown of dietary protein leading to excessive N excretion in faeces and urine. Given the importance of rumen fermentation, it is perhaps not surprising that a great deal of effort has been devoted to investigating methods for manipulating this complex ecosystem.

Some thirteen years ago a paper was presented at the Nottingham Feed Conference on "Developments in rumen fermentation-The scientists view" (Newbold, Stewart and Wallace, 2001); given the passing of time and advances in the subject area it seems appropriate to revisit the topic and specifically to consider:

- Targets for manipulation: i.e. what are the main drivers in terms of altered outputs that are informing research in the area?

- Approaches to manipulation: i.e. what are the prominent approaches to manipulation that are being investigated?

As with the initial article this review is by design a personalised view informed by the opinions and knowledge of the contributors and is not designed, nor should it be viewed, as a complete review of the subject area.

Targets for manipulation

Livestock sustain the livelihood of millions of people in the world in both developing and developed countries. Up to 12% of the world's population is highly dependent on livestock agriculture for their livelihood (Randolph *et al.*, 2007; Thornton *et al.*, 2007). The rapid economic growth observed in some regions of the world has brought increases in income that for a large part of the population translate into higher consumption of animal products per capita. Indeed global consumption of meat is expected to rise from 201 to 334 Mt and milk from 445 to 661 Mt in the 40 years leading to up to 2020 with much of this increase projected to occur in Asia (Steinfeld *et al.*, 2006; FAO, 2009). This increased demand brings challenges in terms of global resource usage and food security.

Possibly the most important challenge facing animal agriculture is direct competition with humans for available nutrients; much of what is currently fed to farm animals could be consumed directly by the human population removing a wasteful trophic level. Pigs and poultry systems have made large gains in feed conversion efficiency over the last 40 years but have become more intensive and dependent on cereals as a major feed ingredient. Similarly, dairy production has been intensified leading to a direct competition with the monogastric livestock in many developed countries. However, the rumen represents an evolutionary advantage for ruminants, since the rumen symbiotic microbes allow ruminants to utilise ligno-cellulose material and to convert non-protein nitrogen into microbial protein. As a result, the efficiency of production of meat, milk and other products from ruminants depends on the basis on which efficiency is considered. It has been estimated that only between 6% and 26% of dietary energy is recovered in ruminant products. However, when calculated as human-edible efficiency (human-edible energy contained in the product divided by human-edible inputs), these values increased to between 52% and 760% recovery dependent on the production system, reflecting the ability of ruminants to utilise fibrous feedstuffs not readily utilised by monogastrics, including man (Gill, Smith and Wilkinson., 2010, Wilkinson., 2011). Indeed the last 13 years has seen an increase in research on the use of agricultural and food industry-residues for feeding ruminants in order to reduce production costs and the environmental burden associated with the accumulation of such by-products (Molina-Alcaide and Yáñez-Ruiz, 2008). Ruminants, when used to transform fibrous feedstuffs produced on land not suitable for primary cropping or by-products of the food industry, can be net contributors to the global supply of human-edible food. Future ruminant production systems will need to capitalize on these important benefits and it is proposed that ruminant agriculture has a key role to play in maintaining and enhancing provision of protein and essential micronutrients (zinc, calcium, iodine, vitamin B_{12} and riboflavin) to man (Scollan *et al.*, 2011).

Unfortunately animal production and in particular ruminant production carries a significant environmental cost both at the local and global level. Although locally this is associated mainly with intensive operations that contaminate the air, land or water with nitrogenous and phosphorous compounds, the global effect is predominantly due to the contribution to emissions of greenhouse gases (GHG), which occurs in both intensive and extensive systems. Global estimates of the contribution of livestock agriculture to total greenhouse gas emissions vary between 9 and 18% of anthropogenic emissions, dependent on whether only direct emissions are accounted for or if emissions associated with the production of feeds, fuel usage, land use change and transport of products etc. are also included in the calculation (Steinfeld *et al.*, 2006). Methane emissions represent between 30 and 50% of the total GHG emitted from the livestock sector with enteric methane from ruminant production systems representing by far the most numerically important source being responsible for circa 80% of the methane emissions from the sector (Steinfeld *et al.*, 2006). Clearly if the ruminant livestock sector is to continue to flourish and grow then new technologies must be developed and implemented that allow it to do so whilst simultaneously decreasing its environmental footprint, produced in a sustainable manner whilst ensuring product quality and safety (Scollan *et al.*, 2011).

In 2001 it was noted that "The targets for manipulation are also changing and no longer can the productivity of the animal be considered in isolation. There is a growing awareness of the health, safety and environmental issues associated with animal agriculture" (Newbold, Stewart and Wallace, 2001), these remarks remain valid in 2014. Indeed in the last few years the term "sustainable intensification" or producing more from less has come into common usage. Whilst we would agree with many that the term "sustainable intensification" is intrinsically contradictory the underlying concept remains valid and we find the definition provided by Smith (2013):

> "The process of delivering more safe, nutritious food per unit of input resource, whilst allowing the current generation to meet its needs without compromising the ability of future generations to meet their own needs"

a useful starting point from which to refine our original statement and from which to base our evaluation of targets and approaches to rumen manipulation. However, perhaps missing from our initial considerations and that of Smith (2013) is the ethical and welfare issues associated with ruminant production. It seems likely that with both the increasing wealth and sophistication of developing markets this may well become an increasing concern. Whilst the nascent debate within developed economies of the need for change in demand side drivers (i.e. lowering meat and milk consumption) as well as production side changes in response to concerns over the role of livestock as a driver of climate change will inevitably drive increased discussion about the ethical and welfare aspect of animal production systems (Ripple *et al.*, 2014).

Approaches to manipulation

The key to understanding and indeed manipulating ruminant production is the rumen. Microbial fermentation in the rumen plays a central role in the ability of ruminants to utilize fibrous substrates. As noted above, however, rumen fermentation also has potential deleterious environmental consequences as it ultimately leads to emission of greenhouse gases and breakdown of dietary protein leading to excessive N excretion in faeces and urine. Whilst fermentation of rapidly degradable substrates can lead to animal welfare concerns if excess acid is formed and can affect the nutritional quality of milk and meat available for human consumption. In 2001 we noted that "There is growing resistance to the use of antibiotic growth promoters within the food chain and the short-term possibility of using genetically modified organisms either by modifying the plants which the animal eats or by introducing modified "superbugs" into the rumen seems unlikely in the face of current consumer concern. Indeed the technologies most likely to be adopted are those that are perceived to be based on natural or green products" (Newbold, Stewart and Wallace, 2001). Again these remarks remain valid however there have been significant advances in developing such approaches in the areas of:

1. An increasing use of molecular biological techniques both to characterise changes in the rumen microbial population in response to additives and to understand the metabolism of rumen microbes thus allowing new additives to be developed.

2. A significant increase in both research and new products based on plant extracts and probiotics designed to increase productivity whilst decreasing greenhouse gas emissions, improving product quality/safety and improving animal welfare.

3. A renewed awareness of the role that the plant plays in rumen fermentation and the use of plant breeding as a means to manipulate rumen fermentation.

4. The developing understanding of the importance of the host in helping determine the microbial population in the rumen, both in terms of the importance of paternal genetics and the importance of early life nutrition in programing the rumen microbial population in later life.

5. The development and implementation of Precision Livestock Farming based on the use of advanced technologies to optimize the contribution of each individual animal.

Improvements in methodology

Traditional studies on rumen microbiology relied on our ability to culture and characterise microorganisms from the rumen (Hobson and Stewart 1997). However whilst significant progress has been made using these techniques over the years, it has been recognised that only a relatively small proportion of the microbes within the rumen are recovered by such techniques leaving us ignorant about the roles and activities of the vast majority of the rumen microbial ecosystem (Edwards *et al.*, 2008). Molecular techniques based on amplification of ribosomal genes have allowed both quantitative and qualitative studies on microbial populations in the rumen to be carried out. Ribosomal genes are believed to be present in all cells; they have highly conserved regions that allow the use of universal primers to amplify the entire microbial ribosomal DNA in a sample (typical 16S rRNA for studying bacteria/archaea and 18S rRNA for studying the fungi and protozoa) and variable regions that allow us to distinguish between different species. Ribosomal genes have been used both to quantify how specific microbial groups respond to rumen manipulation (Belanche *et al.*, 2012) using quantitative PCR (qPCR) and to more qualitatively describe the rumen microbial population and changes induced by manipulation through the characterization of 18/16S rRNA gene pools through massively parallel amplicon sequencing (de la Fuente *et al.*, 2014, Abecia *et al.*, 2014, Pinloche *et al.*, 2013). However, increasingly studies are expanding to consider not only which microbes are present in the rumen but also the functional genes present (metagenomics) and their expression in the rumen (metatranscriptomics) and how this changes in response to rumen manipulation (Morgavi *et al.*, 2013). Modern molecular techniques have also greatly enhanced our understanding of the activity of individual microbial groups in the rumen. The ability to clone and express activities from rumen microbes that were previously uncultivable has provided new insights into rumen function (Newbold *et al.*, 2005, Ricard *et al.*, 2006), and provided new targets for rumen manipulation (Leahy *et al.*, 2013., Wedlock *et al.*, 2013) whilst the ongoing Hungate 1000 project (www.hungate1000.org.nz/) and the associated Global Rumen Census (www.globalrumencensus.org.nz/) promise future advances in which a great deal more is known about the composition of the rumen microbial population and its function.

Plant extracts and probiotics

We have previously reviewed the use of plant extracts to manipulate rumen fermentation both in terms of decreasing methane emissions and improving efficiency of N utilisation (Hart *et al.*, 2008). Bodas *et al.*, (2008) screened 450 plant extracts for their ability to inhibit methane production in *in vitro* incubations of rumen fluid and found that 35 plants extracts decreased methane production by more than 15% *versus* those with corresponding control cultures and, with 6 of these plant additives, the depression in methane production was more than 25%, with no adverse effects on digestion or fermentation. Cieslak *et al* (2013) focused on the mode of action of plant extracts concluding that essential oils, tannins and saponins differed in their mode of action within the rumen and concluded that whilst there was a significant body of work from in vitro studies there was a need for more in vivo and production based studies.

Amongst the various plant extracts that have been investigated for their effect in the rumen, experience with garlic based compounds perhaps helps illustrate both the state of the art and the current constraints that require further research input. Garlic oil is a mix of a large number of different molecules that are found in the plant or occur as the result of changes occurring during oil extraction and processing Although garlic oil is known for a wide variety of therapeutic properties (antiparasitic, insecticidal, anticancer, antioxidant, inmunomodulatory, anti-inflammatory, hypoglycaemic), and its antimicrobial activity against a wide spectrum of gram-positive and gram-negative bacteria is often seen as its most prominent activity and has been thoroughly studied (Reuter *et al.*, 1996), its potential effect on modifying rumen microbial fermentation had not been researched until recently. *In vitro* rumen fluid fermentation trials (Busquet *et al.*, 2005, 2006, Soliva *et al.*, 2011) have shown that garlic oil altered rumen fermentation and decreased methane production. We have shown that a commercially available aqueous allicin extract from garlic had no effect on general rumen fermentation but caused a 94% decrease in methane production, and that this was accompanied by a reduction in the number of methane producing Archaea in the rumen assessed by qPCR (Hart *et al.*, 2008). However, with many additives, the anti-methanogenic activity is short-term as the rumen adapts to overcome the new chemical introduced (McAllister and Newbold, 2008). The same is true for many plant extracts, where effects on fermentation seem to disappear when tested for longer periods of time (Cardozo *et al.*, 2004; Molero *et al.*, 2004; Castillejos *et al.*, 2007). The long-term effect of products based on garlic is not yet known, although relatively short-term animal trials (5-6 weeks) have recorded consistent decreases in methane emission over this period, and an increase in ruminal propionate suggesting that rumen can adapt to find an alternative hydrogen sink (Klevenhusena *et al.*, 2011, Hart *et al.*, 2012). Nevertheless, the lack of long-term trials is a major deficiency in the literature concerning the use of plant extracts to alter rumen function. Similarly, reports of taint in the milk of animals eating wild garlic and onions exist from the 1930s (Babcock, 1938). Whilst it is possible that commercial extracts produced from garlic may not taint milk and meat, the possibility of taint is a very real concern and, unless tested and addressed, will remain a likely barrier to the uptake of any technology based on compounds isolated from garlic or other plant extracts.

Yeast culture

Yeast cultures based on *Saccharomyces cerevisiae* are widely used in ruminant diets. Available products vary widely in both the strain of *S. cerevisiae* used and the number and viability of yeast cells present. We have noted that not all strains of the yeast are capable of stimulating digestion in the rumen (Newbold, McIntosh and Wallace., 1995). Certain strains of *S. cerevisiae* can help prevent the decrease in rumen pH associated with feeding a cereal-based diet and this appears to be associated with a decrease in rumen lactate concentrations (Newbold, McIntosh and Wallace, 1998). Rumen pH is one of the most critical determinants of rumen function particularly for the cellulolytic rumen bacteria which fail to grow at pH 6.0 and below (Stewart, 1977). Rumen pH falls as a result of enhanced fermentation due to increasing concentrate in the diet; this fall inhibits degradation of the fibrous components of the diet and is the cause, in part at least, of the negative associative effects between forages and concentrates. It has been suggested that feed additives based on *S. cerevisiae* could help alleviated this post feeding drop in rumen pH (Williams *et al.*, 1991) resulting in a more stable rumen fermentation (Harrison *et al.*, 1988). Acute rumen acidosis occurs when a ruminant ingests a large quantity of rapidly fermented carbohydrates. The microbial changes in the rumen associated with such an event have been visualized as a spiral in which the availability of rapidly fermentable carbohydrate results in the production of volatile fatty acids by a wide range of rumen microorganisms with an associated drop in rumen pH. Then, in some cases, an overgrowth of *Streptococcus bovis* (facilitated by this organism's ability to uncouple growth from carbohydrate fermentation; Cook and Russell, 1994, Russell, 1998) leads to rapid accumulation of lactic acid and a further drop in pH. As pH declines *lactobacilli* start to predominate, leading to further accumulation of lactic acid and a yet further drop in rumen pH (Russell and Hino, 1985). However, whilst acute acidosis can, and in cases does, lead to death due to associated metabolic acidosis (Dunlop, 1972), sub-acute ruminal acidosis (SARA), also known as chronic or sub-clinical acidosis, is perhaps a more common and well-recognized digestive disorder that is an increasing health problem in many dairy herds. SARA is a disorder of ruminal fermentation that is characterized by extended periods of depressed ruminal pH below 5.5–5.6. As before, this drop in ruminal pH is a result of the breakdown of dietary carbohydrates particularly from cereal grains leading to the production of volatile fatty acids and lactic acid but unlike acute acidosis the rumen pH does not spiral below pH 5 and indeed may recover to above pH 6 later in the feeding cycle. Thus cattle experiencing SARA often do not exhibit any clear overt clinical symptoms with the most common clinical sign associated with SARA being a reduced or erratic feed intake (Krause and Oetzel, 2006, Lean *et al.*, 2013). What is not clear is how yeast prevents the post feeding decline in rumen pH. *S. cerevisiae* had no influence on buffering capacity of rumen fluid (Ryan, 1990) suggesting that pH stabilization is a secondary rather than a direct effect. Similarly it seems unlikely that the yeast directly removed acidic end products from the rumen (Williams *et al.*, 1991) and, although there is some limited evidence that *S. cerevisiae* might out compete the rumen microorganisms for soluble sugars (Williams *et al.*, 1991, Chaucheyras *et al.*, 1996), most studies on the effect of *S. cerevisiae* on rumen pH have focused on effects of the yeast on rumen bacterial population specifically the selective stimulation in growth and metabolism of lactate utilizing bacteria in the rumen such as *Megaspharera elsdenii* and *Selenomonas ruminantium* (Nisbet and Martin, 1991, Chaucheyras *et al.*, 1996, Newbold *et al.*, 1998).

Recently 16S rRNA has been used to characterise the change in the bacterial population within the rumen of cattle fed an acidogenic diet supplemented with live yeast. Samples from the liquid, solid and solid plus liquid phase of the rumen were collected for DNA extraction and the variation in the bacterial community between treatments was assessed by using Terminal Restriction Fragment Length Polymorphism (tRFLP) based on the 16S rRNA gene. There were clear differences between samples taken from the liquid phase of the rumen and those taken from the solid phase, confirming previous observations that a unique microbial population is attached to feed material in the rumen. It was also obvious that a unique and different bacterial population had developed in the rumen of the animals receiving either 0.5 or 5 g/d yeast (Pinloche *et al.*, 2103). Using massively parallel amplicon sequencing we were able to show that Firmicutes accounted for 50% to 60% of the recovered sequences (depending of the treatment), Bacteroidetes (34% to 40%), Proteobacteria (1.2% to 2%), Actinobacteria (0.4% to 1.2%) and Fibrobacteres (0.6% to 1.5%) with 8 minor Phylum (<0.5%). The relative occurrence of Bacteroidetes and Proteobacteria decreased in yeast fed animals; whilst Firmicutes, Fibrobacteres and Actinobacteria increased. When bacteria were classified in functional groupings based on known metabolic activity, a significant decrease in the taxa representing starch consuming bacteria (Mitsuokella), proteolytic bacteria (Prevotella) and an increase in the taxa representing both fibrolytic bacteria (Fibrobacter, Ruminococcus, Eubacterium) and lactic acid utilising bacteria (Megasphaera and Selenomonas) was observed in yeast fed animals (Pinloche *et al.*, 2013). Clearly as we develop and improve our ability to describe the effect of additives on the rumen microbiome we would hope that such information would feed back into the development of more effective manipulation strategies.

Plant based approaches

It is self-evident that the composition of the diet and plants that ruminants consume will alter the rumen microbial ecosystem and its function. However recently there has been increased interest in plant breeding as a means to modify rumen fermentation such as to increase animal productivity whilst reducing the environmental impact of ruminant agriculture (Kingston-Smith *et al.*, 2010, 2013). Lovatt *et al.* (2006) initially suggested that high sugar grasses (HSG) might decrease methane production in the rumen based on in vitro assays. Kim, Newbold and Scollan. (2011) reported that lambs offered HSG had increased dry matter intake and produced the same total methane as those offered a control grass. However, when corrected for dry matter intake lambs offered HSG produced 17% less methane. Staerfl *et al.* (2012) used an energy balance approach to predict that dairy cows offered HSG would have a tendency (P=0.094) to have a lower total daily methane production. Newbold (2010) measured methane emissions in lambs through the growing season (April to June) using the tunnel system described by Murray *et al* (2001). Over the growing period, mean methane emission rates were circa 20% lower for lambs grazing the HSG sward than for those grazing a control sward (8.0 and 10.5 l/lamb/d, respectively; *P*=0.039). Daily live-weight gain was also greater for lambs grazing HSG (152 vs 108 g/animal/d; P<0.01), therefore methane emission reduction per kg live-weight gain was greater than on a per animal basis weight gain. However these experimental results are at odds with the modelling approaches used by Ellis *et al.* (2012) who concluded that based on a dynamic model of rumen function, HSG would have either no effect or increase methane emissions from the rumen and that methane emissions, relative to gross energy intake and g/kg milk, would be reduced by feeding HSG, only if the dry matter intake of cows offered HSG was elevated sufficiently. Perhaps some of this disagreement might explained by recent results (Newbold, unpublished) that suggest that the reduction in methane emissions in animals fed HSG does not seem to be related to the water soluble energy concentration and that other changes in plant chemistry and structure might be important. Indeed Kingston-Smith *et al.*, (2008) have suggested that in grazing animals plant material entering the rumen is not an inert substrate and plant enzymes and stress reactions might influence microbial colonisation of plant material and subsequently rumen fermentation (Kingston Smith *et al.*, 2013)

Host driven effects on the rumen

Evidence is mounting that the host itself might also have an effect on the rumen microbial population (Pacheco, Waghorn and Janssen., 2014). Indeed it is now apparent that within a flock sheep of the same breed on the same diet some animals can be segregated into 'low' or 'high' methane producers (Pinares-Patiño *et al.* 2011) and that to an extent this is heritable (Pinares-Patiño *et al.* 2013). The mechanisms by which the host might control the rumen microbial population remain unknown but factors such as modifying gene expression of the rumen epithelium (Penner *et al.* 2011) and possible variation in rumen outflow or volume (Pinares-Patiño *et al.*2003, 2007, Goopy *et al.* 2014) have been suggested.

In addition to heritable host factors we have also recently investigated the possible role of early life nutrition on microbial population structure and function in adult ruminants. During rumen development, in young ruminants ingested microbes colonise and establish in a defined and progressive sequence (Hobson and Stewart, 1997). Methanogenic archaea and cellulolytic bacteria have been found in the undeveloped rumen of lambs well before the ingestion of solid feed begins (2-4 days) and reach levels similar to those in adult animals around 10 days after birth (Fonty *et al.*, 1987; Morvan *et al.*, 1994). The coexistence of the host and microbial gut communities is clearly immunologically driven, and we are only beginning to understand the complex ways in which they adapt to each other (Winkler *et al.*, 2007, Wedlock *et al.*, 2013).

A recent study of the evolution of mammals and their gut microbes showed that bacterial communities co-diversified with their hosts being mainly influenced by animal species and diet preference, but with high bacterial-host specificity (Ley *et al.*, 2008). Host-level selection of specific members of a microbiota has been demonstrated under laboratory conditions by reciprocal transplantations of gut microbiota from one host species to germ-free recipients of a different species: Groups of bacteria were expanded or contracted in the recipient host to resemble its original gut microbiota (Rawls *et al.*, 2006). Human based studies have shown that the microbial population within the gut is remarkably stable throughout adult life (Faith *et al.*, 2013). Thompson, Wang and Holmes (2008) suggested that the gut environment during postnatal development had a long-term impact on gut community structure, whilst Kerr *et al.*, 2014 suggested that the effects of early life events on the gut microflora, are fundamental in shaping the microbial consortia in the gut throughout life. We have reported that a simple change in nutritional regime (forage vs. concentrate) applied early in life of lambs modified the bacterial population colonizing the rumen and that the effect persists over 4 months (Yáñez-Ruiz *et al.*, 2010). Waddams *et al.* (unpublished) have shown that treating lambs with chloroform (a potent inhibitor of methanogensis) from birth up until weaning had significant effects on methane production and rumen function 4 months after the chloroform treatment stopped and there were still indications of altered rumen function 12 months after the treatment ceased. Abecia *et al* (2014) working with goats found that treating kids and their does with bromochloromethane during the weaning period modified the archaeal community composition colonizing the rumen and although not all the effects persisted after weaning some less abundant archaeal groups remained different in treated and control 4 months after the treatment stopped. Clearly there is a need for more research in this area but if the concept that additives used in early life can affect rumen function in adult life can be confirmed then it will fundamentally change our approach to rumen manipulation.

Precision livestock farming

Precision Livestock Farming – the use of advanced technologies to optimize the contribution of each individual animal – is based in the electronic identification of each individual animal, as well as the usage of automatic feeders and machinery able to measure the animal performance and health (e.g. milk production, lameness and welfare). Therefore, the farmer can have quantitative data about the performance and wellbeing of each animal in real time. The goal of this farming system is to allow a precision feeding based on the "supply of the right nutrient to the right animal, at the right concentration and timing" in order to maximize their efficiency. Considering that the implementation of most of the rumen manipulation alternatives described above represent a substantial cost for the farmer, precision farming could help to implement them and to maximize their potential.

Conclusion

New ways by which the rumen microbes might be manipulated continue to be identified with a growing awareness of the interaction of rumen microbes, the host and the plants the host eats, whilst the targets for manipulation continue to be refined by the changing societal views and concerns regarding the role of ruminant livestock within food production systems and the often contradictory requirements of the sustainable intensification agenda.

References

Abecia, L., Waddams, K.E., Martínez-Fernandez, G., Martín-García, A.I., Ramos-Morales, E., Newbold, C.J. and Yáñez-Ruiz, D.R. . (2014) An antimethanogenic nutritional intervention in early life of ruminants modifies ruminal colonization by Archaea. *Archaea.* **6**; 2014:841463. doi: 10.1155/2014/841463.

Babcock, C.J. (1938) Feed Flavors in Milk and Milk Products. *Journal of Dairy Science,* **21** : 661-668.

Belanche, A., Doreau, M., Edwards, J.E., Moorby, J.M., Pinloche, E. and Newbold, C.J. (2012) Shifts in the rumen microbiota due to the type of carbohydrate and level of protein ingested by dairy cattle are associated with changes in rumen fermentation. *Journal of Nutrition*; **142**, 1684-1692.

Bodas, R., Lopez, S., Fernández, M., García-González, R., Rodríguez, A.B., Wallace, R.J. and González, J.S. (2008) In vitro screening of the potential of numerous plant species as antimethanogenic feed additives for ruminants *Animal Feed Science and Technology*, **145**, 245-258.

Busquet, M., Calsamiglia, S., Ferret, A., Carro, M.D. and Kamel, C. (2005) Effect of garlic oil and four of its compounds on rumen microbial fermentation. *Journal of Dairy Science*, **88**, 4393–4404.

Busquet, M., Calsamiglia, S., Ferret, A. and Kamel, C. (2006) Plant extracts affect in vitro rumen microbial fermentation. *Journal of Dairy Science*, **89**, 761–771.

Cardozo, P.W., Calsamiglia, S., Ferret, A. and Kamel, C. (2004) Effects of natural plant extracts on ruminal protein degradation and fermentation profiles in continuous culture. *Journal of Animal Science*, **82**, 3230–3236.

Castillejos, L., Calsamiglia, S., Ferret, A. and Losa, R. (2007) Effects of dose and adaptation time of a specific blend of essential oil compounds on rumen fermentation. *Animal Feed Science and Technology*, **132**, 186–201.

Chaucheyras, F., Fonty, G., Bertin, G., Salmon, J.M. and Gouet, P. (1996) Effects of a strain of Saccharomyces cerevisiae (Levucell SC1), a microbial additive for ruminants, on lactate metabolism in vitro. *Canadian Journal of Microbiology,* **42**: 927-933

Cieslak, A., Szumacher-Strabel, M., Stochmal, A. and Oleszek, W. (2013) Plant components with specific activities against rumen methanogens. *Animal,* **7**. 253-265.

Cook, G.M., and Russell, J.B. (1994) Energy-spilling reactions of *Streptococcus bovis* and resistance of its membrane to proton conductance. *Applied and Environmental Microbiology,* **60**, 1942–1948.

de la Fuente, G., Belanche, A., Girwood, S.E., Pinloche, E,, Wilkinson, T. and Newbold, C.J. (2014) Pros and cons of ion-torrent next generation sequencing versus terminal restriction fragment length polymorphism T-RFLP for studying the rumen bacterial community. *PLoS One.* 9: e101435.

Dunlop, R.H, (1972) Pathogenesis of ruminant lactic acidosis. *Advances in Veterinary Science & Comparative Medicine,* **16,** 259-302

Edwards, J.E., Huws, S.A., Kim, E.J., Lee, M.R.F., Kingston-Smith, A.H. and Scollan, N.D. (2008) Advances in microbial ecosystem concepts and their consequences for ruminant digestion. *Animal,* **2**, 653-660.

Ellis, J.L., Dijkstra, J., France, J., Parsons, A. J., Edwrads, G. R. Rasmussen, S., Kebraeb, E. and Bannink, A. (2012) Effect of high-sugar grasses on methane emissions simulated using a dynamic model. *Journal of Dairy Science,* **95**, 272-285.

Faith, J.J., Guruge, J.L, Charbonneau, M., Subramanian, S., Seedorf, H., Goodman, A.L., Clemente, J.C., Knight, R., Heath, A.C., Leibel, R.L.,, Rosenbaum, M., and Gordon, J. (2013) The long-term stability of the human gut microbiota. *Science,* **341** (6141), 1237439.

FAO (2009) *The State of Food and Agriculture - Livestock in the Balance.* Food and Agriculture Organisation of the United Nations, Rome, Italy.

Fonty, G., Gouet,P., Jouany, J.P. and Senaud, J. (1987) Establishment of the microflora and anaerobic fungi in the rumen of lambs. *Journal of General Microbiology,* **133**, 835–1843.

Goopy, J.P., Donaldson, A, Hegarty, R, Vercoe, P..E, Haynes, F., Barnett, M. and Oddy, V.H. (2014) Low-methane yield sheep have smaller rumens and shorter rumen retention time. *The British Journal of Nutrition,* **111**, 578–585.

Kerr, C.A.,Grice D.M., Tran,C.D., Bauer, D.C., Li, D., Hendry,P. and Hannan, G.N. (2014) Early life events influence whole-of-life metabolic health via gut microflora and gut permeability *Critical Reviews in Microbiology,* Ahead of Print : doi:10.3109/1040841X.2013.837863

Kim, E J., Newbold, C.J. and Scollan, N. D. (2011) Effect of water-soluble carbohydrate in fresh forage on growth and methane production by growing lambs. *Advances in Animal Biosciences,* **2**. 270 (abstract).

Kingston-Smith, A,H., Davies,T.E,, Edwards, J.E. and Theodorou, M.K. (2008) From plants to animals; the role of plant cell death in ruminant herbivores. *Journal of Experimental Botany,* **59,** 521-532.

Kingston-Smith, A.H., Edwards, J.E., Huws, S.A., Kim, E.J. and Abberton, M. (2010) Plant-based strategies towards minimising 'livestock's long shadow'. *Proceedings of The Nutrition Society,* **69**, 613-620.

Kingston-Smith, A.H., Marshall, A.H. and Moorby, J.M (2013)Breeding for genetic improvement of forage plants in relation to increasing animal production with reduced environmental footprint. *Animal,* **7**, 79-88.

Kingston-Smith, A.H., Davies, T.E., Rees Stevens, P., and Mur, L.A. (2013) Comparative metabolite fingerprinting of the rumen system during colonisation of three forage grass (Lolium perenne L.) varieties. *PLoS One.;***8**, e82801.

Klevenhusena, F., Duval, S., Zeitz, J.O., Kreuzer, M. and Soliva, C.R. (2011) Diallyl disulphide and lovastatin: effects on energy and protein utilisation in, as well as methane emission from, sheep. *Archives of Animal Nutrition*, **65**, 255-66.

Krause, K.M. and Oetzel, G.R. (2006) Understanding and preventing subacute ruminal acidosis in dairy herds : A review *Animal Feed Science and Technology*, **126**, 215-236,

Gill, M., Smith, P. and Wilkinson, J.M. (2010). Mitigating climate change: the role of domestic livestock. *Animal*, **4**, 323-333.

Harrison, G.A., Hemken, R.W,, Dawson, K.A., Harmon, R.J. and Barker, K.B. (1988) Influence of addition of yeast culture supplement to diets of lactating cows on ruminal fermentation and microbial populations. *Journal of Dairy Science*, **71**, 2967-2975.

Hart, K.J., Yanez-Ruiz, D.R., Duval, S.M., McEwan, N.R. and Newbold, C.J. (2008) Plant extracts to manipulate rumen fermentation. *Animal Feed Science and Technology*, **147**, 8-35.

Hart, K.J., Easton, G.L., Worgan, H.J. and Newbold, C.J (2012) The effect of Javanol, Allicin, and probiotic yeast on in vivo methane production, nitrogeon retention and rumen bacterial diversity in store lambs. In *Gut Microbiota: Friend or Foes*. Proceedings of the 8th INRA-Rowett Symposium on Gut Microbiology (available at https://colloque4.inra.fr/inra_rowett_2012/Post-congress-materials)

Hobson, P.N. and Stewart, C.S. (1997) *The Rumen Microbial Ecosystem*. 2nd edition. Springer, New York.

Leahy, S.C., Kelly, W.J., Ronimus, R.S., Wedlock, N., Altermann, E. and Attwood, G.T. (2013) Genome sequencing of rumen bacteria and archaea and its application to methane mitigation strategies. *Animal*, **7**, 235-243.

Lean, I.J., Westwood, C.T., Golder, H.M. and Vermunt, J.J. (2013) Impact of nutrition on lameness and claw health in cattle. *Livestock Science* **156**, 71-87.

Ley, R.E., Hamady, M., Lozupone, C., Turnbaugh, P.J., Ramey, R.R., Bircher, J.S., Schlegel, M.L., Tucker, T.A., Schrenzel, M.D., Knight, R. and Gordon, J. (2008) Evolution of mammals and their gut microbes. *Science* **20**, 1647-1651.

Lovett, D.K., McGillowey, D., Bortoozz, A., Hawkins, M., Calland, J, Flynn, B and OMarra, F.P. (2006) *In vitro* fermentation patterns and methane production as influenced by cultivar and season of harvest of *Lolium perenne* L *Grass and Forage Science* **61**, 9-21.

McAllister, T. and Newbold, C.J. (2008) Redirecting rumen fermentation to reduce methanogenesis. *Australian Journal of Experimental Agriculture* **48**, 7-13.

Molero, R., Ibars, M., Calsamiglia, S., Ferret, A. and Losa, (2004). Effects of a specific blend of essential oil compounds on dry matter and crude protein degradability in heifers fed diets with different forage to concentrate ratios. *Animal Feed Science and Technology* **114**, 91–104.

Molina-Alcaide, E. and Yáñez-Ruiz, D.R. (2008) Potential use of olive by-products in ruminant feeding: A review. *Animal Feed Science and Technology*, **147**, 247-264.

Morgavi, D.P., Kelly, W.J., Janssen, P.H. and Attwood, G.T. (2013) Rumen microbial (meta) genomics and its application to ruminant production. *Animal* **7**, 184–201.

Morvan, B., Dore, J., Rieu-Lesme, F., Foucat, L., Fonty, G. and Gouet, P. (1994) Establishment of hydrogen-utilizing bacteria in the rumen of the newborn lamb. *FEMS Microbiology Letters* **117**, 249-256.

Murray, P.J., Gill, E., Balsdon, S.L. and Jarvis, S.C. (2001) A comparison of methane emissions from sheep grazing pastures with differing management intensities. *Nutrient Cycling in Agroecosystems,* **60,** 93-97.

Newbold, C.J. (2010) Ruminant Nutrition Regimes to Reduce methane & Nitrogen Emmissions. DEFRA Final Project Report available at: http://randd.defra.gov.uk/Default.aspx?Menu= Menu&Module=More&Location=None&Completed=0&ProjectID=14952

Newbold, C.J., McIntosh, F.M. and Wallace R.J. (1995) Different strains of Saccharomyces cerevisiae differ in their effects on ruminal bacteria in vitro and in sheep. *Journal of Animal Science,* **73,** 1811-1818

Newbold ,C.J., McIntosh, F.M. and Wallace, R.J. (1998) Changes in the microbial population of a rumen-simulating fermenter in response to yeast culture. *Canadian Journal of Animal Science.* **78,** 241- 244.

Newbold, C.J., Stewart, C.S. and Wallace, R.J. (2001) Developments in rumen fermentation-The scientists view. In *Recent Advances in Animal Nutrition - 2001.* (Garnsworthy, P.C. and Wiseman, J Eds) pp 251-279, Nottingham University Press, Nottingham.

Newbold, C.J., McEwan, N.R., Calza, R.E., Chareyron, E.N., Duval, S.M., Eschenlauer, S.C., McIntosh, F.M., Nelson, N., Travis, A.J. and Wallace, R.J. (2005) An NAD(+)-dependent glutamate dehydrogenase cloned from the ruminal ciliate protozoan, Entodinium caudatum. *FEMS Microbiology Letters* **247**,113-21.

Nisbet, D.J. and Martin, S.A. (1991) The effect of Saccharomyces cerevisiae culture on lactate utilization by the ruminal bacterium Selenomonas ruminantium. *Journal of Animal Science,* **69,** 4628-4633.

Pacheco, D., Waghorn, G. and Janssen, P.H. (2014) Decreasing methane emissions from ruminants grazing forages: a fit with productive and financial realities? *Animal Production Science,* **54,** 1141–1154

Penner, G.B., Steele, M.A., Aschenbach, J.R. and McBride, B.W. (2011) Ruminant nutrition symposium: molecular adaptation of ruminal epithelia to highly fermentable diets. *Journal of Animal Science,* **89,** 1108–1119.

Pinares-Patiño, C.S., Ebrahimi, E.H., McEwan, J.C., Dodds, K.G., Clark, H. and Luo, D. (2011) Is rumen retention time implicated in sheep differences in methane emission? *Proceedings of the New Zealand Society of Animal Production,* **71,** 219–222.

Pinares-Patiño, C.S,, Ulyatt, M.J., Lassey, K.R., Barry, T.N. and Holmes, C.W. (2003) Rumen function and digestion parameters associated with differences between sheep in methane emissions when fed chaffed lucerne hay. *The Journal of Agricultural Science,* **140,** 205–214.

Pinares-Patiño, C.S., Waghorn, G.C., Machmüller, A., Vlaming, B., Molano, G., Cavanagh, A. and Clark, H. (2007) Methane emissions and digestive physiology of non-lactating dairy cows fed pasture forage. *Canadian Journal of Animal Science,* **87,** 601–613.

Pinares-Patiño, C.S., Hickey, S.M., Young, E.A, Dodds, K.G, MacLean, S, Molano, G, Sandoval, E, Kjestrup, H, Harland, R, Hunt, C, Pickering, N.K. and McEwan J.C. (2013) Heritability estimates of methane emissions from sheep. *Animal,* **7**,316-321.

Pinloche E, McEwan N, Marden, J.P, Bayourthe C, Auclair E and Newbold C.J. (2013) The effects of a probiotic yeast on the bacterial diversity and population structure in the rumen of cattle. *PLoS One.* **8**:e67824.

Randolph, T. F., Schelling, E., Grace, D., Nicholson, C. F., Leroy, J. L., Cole, D. C., Dentment, M. W., Omore, A., Zinsstag, J. and Ruel, M. (2007) Invited Review: Role of livestock in human nutrition and health for poverty reduction in developing countries. *Journal of Animal Science*, **85**, 2788-2800.

Rawls, J.F., Mahowald, M.A, Ley, R.E. and Gordon, J. (2006) Reciprocal gut microbiota transplants from zebrafish and mice to germ-free recipients reveal host habitat selection *Cell* **127**, 423-433

Reuter, H.D., Koch, H.P. and Lawson, L.D. (1996) Therapeutic effects and applications of garlic and its preparations. In: Garlic. The science and therapeutic application of *Allium sativum* L. and related species pp 135-212. (Edited by Koch HP, Lawson LD) Williams and Wilkins, Baltimore.

Ricard, G., McEwan, N.R,, Dutilh, B.E., Jouany, J.P, Macheboeuf, D., Mitsumori, M., McIntosh, F.M., Michalowski, T., Nagamine, T., Nelson, N., Newbold, C.J., Nsabimana, E., Takenaka, A., Thomas, N.A., Ushida, K., Hackstein, J.H. and Huynen, M.A. (2006) . Horizontal gene transfer from Bacteria to rumen Ciliates indicates adaptation to their anaerobic, carbohydrates-rich environment. *BMC Genomics*, **7**, 22.

Ripple, W.J., Smith, P., Haberl, H., Montzka, S.A., McAlpine , C. and Boucher, DH. (2014) Ruminants, climate change and climate policy *Nature Climate Change*, **4**, 2-5.

Russell, J.B. (1998) Strategies that ruminal bacteria use to handle excess carbohydrate *Journal of Animal Science,* **76**, 1955-1963.

Russell, J.B., and Hino, T (1985) Regulation of lactate production in Streptococcus bovis : A spiraling effect that contributes to rumen acidosis. *Journal of Dairy Science*, **68**, 1712-1721.

Ryan, J.P. (1990) The suggestion that the yeast cell Saccharomyces cerevisiae may absorb sufficient hydrogen ions to increase ruminal fluid pH is untenable *Biochemical Society Transactions*, **18**, 350- 351.

Scollan N D, Greenwood, P L Newbold C J, Yáñez D R, Shingfield K J Wallace, R J and Hocquette J F (2011) Future research priorities for animal production in a changing world *Animal Production Science*, **51**, 1-5.

Smith P (2013) Delivering food security without increasing pressure on land. *Global Food Security*, **2**, 18–23.

Soliva, C.R., Amelchanka, S.L., Duval, S.M., and Kreuzer, M. (2011) Ruminal methane inhibition potential of various pure compounds in comparison with garlic oil as determined with a rumen simulation technique (Rusitec). *British Journal of Nutrition*, **106**, 14-22.

Staerfl, S.M., Zeitz, J.O., Amelchanka, S.L., Kalber, Kreuzer, M. and Leiber, F. (2013) Comparison of the milk fatty acid composition of dairy cows fed high-sugar ryegrass, low-sugar ryegrass, or maize. *Dairy Science and Technology,* **93**, 201-210.

Steinfeld, H., Gerber, P., Wassenaar, T., Castel, V., Rosales, M. and de Haan, C. (2006). *Livestock's Long Shadow: Environmental Issues and Options.* Food and Agriculture Organization (FAO), Rome.

Stewart, C.S. (1977) Factors Affecting the Cellulolytic Activity of Rumen Contents Applied and *Environmental Microbiology*, **33**, 497-502.

Thornton, P., Herrero, M., Freeman, A., Mwai, O., Rege, E., Jones, P. & McDermott, J. (2007) Vulnerability, climate change and livestock – research opportunities and challenges for poverty alleviation. Journal of *SAT Journal Agricultural Research*, 4, 23pp. doi 10.3914/ICRISAT.0109

Thompson, C. L., Wang, B. and Holmes, J. (2008) The immediate environment during postnatal development has long-term impact on gut community structure in pigs. *The ISME Journal*, **2**, 739–748.

Wedlock, D.N., Janssen, P.H., Leahy, S.C., Shu, D. and Buddle B.M.(2013) Progress in the development of vaccines against rumen methanogens. *Animal*, **7**, 244-252.

Wilkinson, J.M. (2011) Re-defining efficiency of feed use by livestock *Animal*, **5**, 1014-1022.

Williams, P.E.V., Tait, C.A.G., Innes, G.M. and Newbold, C.J. (1991) Effects of the inclusion of yeast culture (Saccharomyces cerevisiae plus growth medium) in the diet of dairy cows on milk yield and forage degradation and fermentation patterns in the rumen of sheep and steers. *Journal of Animal Science,* **69**, 3016-3026.

Winkler, P., Ghadimi, D., Schrezenmeir, J., Kraehenbuhl, J.P. (2007). Molecular and cellular basis of microflorahost interactions. *Journal of Nutrition* **137**, 756S-72S.

Yáñez-Ruiz, D.R., Macías, B., Pinloche, E. and Newbold, C.J. (2010) The persistence of bacterial and methanogenic archaeal communities residing in the rumen of young lambs. *FEMS Microbiology Ecology*, **72** 272-278.

6

Dairy Calf and Heifer Rearing for Optimum Lifetime Performance

ALEX BACH

Department of Ruminant Production, IRTA, 08140 Caldes de Montbui, Spain and ICREA, 08007 Barcelona, Spain

Introduction

Feeding methods and management practices applied to today's dairy replacements will influence the performance (and economic returns) of dairy herds in 2016 and onwards. Due to this relatively long time lag, most producers and dairy consultants tend devote less-than-desirable efforts and attention to calf and heifer rearing. In contrast to the situation in lactating cows, where management is typically based on records of milk yield, milk composition, feed intake, body condition, etc., heifers are managed based on "feeling" rather than being based on methodical data collection and record keeping. This chapter will review several nutritional aspects aimed at improving performance of calves and heifers, minimizing health disorders, and setting the stage to achieve first calving at 23-24 months of age with a body weight (BW) above 650 kg (before calving), which should result in optimum milk production and longevity.

Setting the stage for the future

Nowadays, it is clear that nutrient supply and hormonal signals at specific windows during development (both pre- and early post-natal) may exert permanent changes in the metabolism of humans (Fall, 2011), as well as changes in performance, body composition, and metabolic function of the offspring of livestock (Wu *et al.*, 2006) through processes generically referred to as foetal programming and metabolic imprinting. Thus, it is likely that today's cow, with high milk yield but also reproductive and metabolic challenges, is not only a consequence of genetic selection, but also the result of the way her dam was fed and the way she was fed early after birth as a calf and later as a heifer (Bach, 2012).

The first weeks of life seem to have long-lasting consequences on the physiological function of neonates. The pioneering work of McCance (1962) illustrated that

79

limit-feeding rats during the first 21 d of life resulted in a lifetime programming of growth pattern that was lesser than that of rats fed properly. More interestingly, when the same dietary restriction was applied for 21 d but at a more advanced age, the intervention had no lasting effect because the underfed rats showed compensatory growth gains when re-fed at normal levels (Figure 1). In dairy cattle, there is some evidence that the nutritional level of the first 2 months of life also exerts long-term effects expressed as improvements in milk yield (Davis Rincker *et al.*, 2008; Margerison *et al.*, 2014). Even the type of calving seems to exert an effect on calves. Barrier *et al.* (2012) reported a greater mortality risk to weaning and to first service in the live-born heifers that experienced moderate difficulty at birth compared with heifers born to unproblematic calvings.

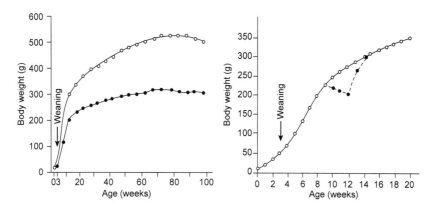

Figure 1. Effect of a 3-week feed restriction applied at two different stages of development on growth in rats (Adapted from McCance, 1962).

The analysis of a dataset including data from 900 animals raised in a contract heifer operation in Spain and followed into 3 different dairy herds revealed a significant positive relationship between average daily gain (ADG) during the first 65 d of age (with ADG ranging from 0.37 to 1.12 kg/d) and future milk yield (Bach and Ahedo, 2008). Later, Bach (2012) conducted a meta-analysis and concluded that about 225 kg of additional milk in the first lactation could be expected for each additional 100 g/d of growth during the first 2 months of life. Furthermore, two recent prospective studies indicate that growth rate is positively correlated with survivability to second lactation (Bach, 2011; Heinrichs and Heinrichs, 2011). Therefore, providing the necessary nutrition to sustain rapid growth rates (>750 g/d) during the first 2 months, should result not only in more efficient (and economically better, as discussed later), but also in more effective (greater milk performance) heifer rearing.

Nourishing the calf

Liquid feeding

The first action to perform is to ensure that the new-born calf receives adequate amounts of antibodies and nutrients to avoid falling ill in early stages of life. Both, immunity and nutrients should be provided though adequate amounts of good quality colostrum. Despite the fact that colostrum is more commonly considered a source of immunity than a source of nutrients, the first nutrients that new-born calves consume are derived from colostrum. In addition to nutrients, colostrum is also rich in growth factors and hormones, and thus it could also have a potential impact on future performance. The pioneering work by DeNise et al. (1989) demonstrated a positive and significant relationship between plasma IgG concentrations and future milk production of calves that were allowed to suckle their dams for the first 24 h of life. DeNise et al. (1989) acknowledged that this association was probably not due to IgG directly, and suggested that it was probably linked to *other factors* in colostrum that could influence subsequent production. An example of the importance of *other factors* can be found in the study by Hough et al. (1990). These authors nourished cows during the last third of pregnancy to 100 or 60% of their nutrient requirements. Interestingly, despite the fact that maternal nutrition did not affect colostral IgG concentrations, calves born to non-restricted cows that received colostrum from restricted dams tended to have lower serum IgG concentrations at 24 h of life than those receiving colostrum from well-nourished cows. Tri-iodothyronine participates in IgG absorption at the intestinal level (Boland et al., 2008), and lower colostral tri-iodothyronine concentrations exhibited by the nutrient-restricted mothers, compared with control dams, could be one of the reasons why serum IgG concentrations decreased. An example of the potential long-term effects of colostrum was reported by Faber et al. (2005), who described a 10% increase in mature equivalent milk production during the first lactation, and 15% during the second lactation, in cows that received 4 l instead of 2 l of colostrum at birth. The long-term effects of colostrum feeding are most likely related to important constituents, such as IGF-I, IGF-II, insulin, growth hormone, epidermal growth factor, leptin, and prolactin. These hormones could participate in lactocrine mechanisms to elicit modifications of several hormonal axes in the calf.

After birth, once colostrum has been provided, the calf should be transferred into an individual hutch without possibility of licking other calves. Nutrition at this age should be based on water, whole milk or milk replacer (MR), and a starter. Water should be made available to calves at all times. Milk or MR does not reach the rumen (it goes directly into the omasum), and thus only water will provide the necessary moist environment that bacteria need to colonize the rumen. Insufficient provision of water limits starter intake and thus growth. Calves need to consume, in addition to milk or MR, 4 to 6 l of water for every kg of starter.

Milk or MR provides the main source of nutrients for young calves. Feeding whole milk is usually not economic and may pose problems of consistency of nutrient composition. On the other hand, MR represents an economic advantage and has a consistent composition (if prepared carefully). However, MR provides less energy to the calf than whole milk, thus growth performance might be comprised. A good MR should contain 250 g of crude protein (CP)/kg and 190 g of fat/kg. Typically, MR are fed at a dilution rate of 125 g/kg (similar to the solids content of milk). However, ADG can be doubled by following intensive liquid feeding programmes that consist of feeding MR up to a 17% dilution and offering up to 8 l/d of MR. This type of programme requires good monitoring of starter intake to ensure that animals do not show reduced growth rate after weaning. Ideally, intensive feeding programs should use a high-quality MR with 270 g of CP/kg and about 150-170 g of fat/kg. It is important that during cold weather, MR is fed at a greater concentration (i.e., dilution rate 150 g/kg instead of 125 g/kg) to provide additional energy to calves to cover the increased maintenance requirements.

An "ideal" feeding programme for calves would consist of feeding 6 l/d at 125 g/kg dilution rate (in winter dilution rate can be changed to 150 g/kg). Feeding 8 l/d may compromise intake of starter (Bach *et al.*, 2013b) and if MR is offered only twice daily, it may foster insulin resistance in calves (Bach *et al.*, 2013a). At the age of 56 d, calves can (and should) be pre-weaned by reducing the offer of liquid feeding to only one 3-l dose a day, and completely weaned at 63 d. It is expected, that calves would be consuming about 1.8 kg/d of starter at 56 d and more than 2.5 kg/d at 63 d, which should ensure that they could maintain a growth rate above 1 kg/d after weaning. Another alternative involves the use of automatic nourishing machines that allow progressive weaning by reducing MR allowances in a more gradual fashion (Khan *et al.*, 2007; Roth *et al.*, 2009).

Attaining maximum growth with solid feed

Because increasing plane of nutrition (and growth) early in life has been correlated with improved milk yield (Bach, 2012) and also with changes in gut microbial diversity and immune response of calves (Ballou, 2013; Malmuthuge *et al.*, 2013; Hengst *et al.*, 2013; Obeidat *et al.*, 2014), maximizing nutrient intake of calves must be ensured. If rapid growth (>750 g/d) early in life is sought, feeding increased amounts of milk is necessary. However, calves fed high milk allowances tend to struggle during transition onto solid feed, and part of the growth advantage achieved before weaning may be lost due to (1) diminished consumption of nutrients, and (2) reduced digestibility. Early consumption of dry feed fosters early rumen microbial development, resulting in greater rumen metabolic activity (Anderson *et al.*, 1987). Thus, the high level of MR offered to calves in enhanced-growth feeding programmes, may delay the start of dry feed consumption and, consequently, may delay rumen development. In fact, duodenal microbial flow of calves following an enhanced-growth feeding programme was lower than that of calves fed conventionally (Terré et al., 2007), suggesting the existence of a poor rumen microflora population that may result in decreased rumen metabolic activity, and may negatively affect starter digestibility at weaning.

Promoting solid feed intake is of crucial importance when feeding more generous milk allowances to calves. Starter feed consumption can be improved by including 'palatable' ingredients in the formulation of the starter. Miller-Cushon et al. (2014) evaluated the palatability of several energy and protein ingredients commonly used in starters and concluded that corn gluten feed and corn gluten meal should be avoided, and that wheat, sorghum, maize and soyabean meal should be prioritized to increase palatability of starters. Oats, which are commonly included in starters, were found to have low palatability, and thus their inclusion in formulation of starter should not be forced. In terms of nutrients, a good starter should contain 180 g of CP/kg and 13.4 MJ/kg of metabolisable energy (ME), although starters containing 200 g of CP/kg or more may have some benefits immediately after weaning when rearing calves in intensified milk regimes to provide sufficient metabolisable protein and ensure amino acids do not limit growth.

Several recent studies (Khan, et al, 2011; Castells et al., 2012, Castells et al., 2013; Montoro et al., 2013) have shown that another effective method to encourage solid feed intake of calves, contrary to what has been traditionally recommended, is to provide ad libitum access to poor quality (nutritionally) chopped straw or chopped grass hay. In the last century, it was believed that feeding a fibre source to young dairy calves was necessary because it improved rumen health and that if no forage was provided to calves, low fibre content of the complete starter should be avoided (Jahn et al., 1970; Thomas and Hinks, 1982). Later, in the 1970s, the concept of textured starter was introduced (Warner et al., 1973). It was assumed that with textured starters no additional feeding of forage was needed. Furthermore, the use of fibrous feeds has been discouraged since then because of the limited fibre digestion during the pre-weaning period, and because the potential accumulation of undigested forage material in the rumen could decrease voluntary intake of concentrate (Drackley, 2008). However, several authors (Kincaid, 1980; Thomas and Hinks, 1992; Phillips 2004; Suárez et al., 2007; Castells et al., 2012) reported either an increase in starter intake or no effect on total feed consumption with inclusion of dietary forage. Castells et al. (2012) offered a pelleted starter feed containing 180 g of NDF/kg and 195 g of CP/kg in conjunction with different sources of chopped forage to young dairy calves, and reported that feeding chopped grass hay or straw improved solid feed intake (by more than 23%) and rate of growth, without impairing nutrient digestibility and gain to feed ratio. In contrast, when the forage fed was alfalfa hay, these benefits were not observed.

There have been concerns, however, about the potential confounding effects of gut fill when introducing forages to young calves (if gut fill increases, BW is artificially increased). Several studies (Hill *et al.*, 2008) have argued that feeding forage (hay and straw) to pre-weaned dairy heifers reduces starter and overall dry matter consumption. In the studies by Castells *et al.* (2012, 2013), when calves were fed ad libitum chopped alfalfa hay, forage intake was 14% of total solid feed intake, whereas when calves were offered chopped oat straw, forage consumption did not exceed 4% of total solid feed intake. Previous studies have shown that high proportions of forage in the diet of calves drastically increase gut fill, but not when forage intake is less than 5% of the total solid diet. For instance, Stobo *et al.* (1966) limit-fed a starter feed and offered hay at different proportions (from 4 to 61% of total solid feed intake) and reported an increase in gut fill from 23.5 to 32.5% of total BW. Similarly, Strozinski and Chandler (1971) and Jahn *et al.* (1970) reported an increase in gut fill from about 7-10% to 20-24% when feeding 0 or 5% to a 60-90% inclusion of hay in the diet of calves. More recently, Castells (2013) conducted a meta-analysis and concluded that there was no difference in gut fill between calves with no access to forage and calves consuming forage up to 5% of total solid feed consumption. Thus, it can be safely concluded that when forage consumption is less than 5% of total solid feed intake, gut fill is negligible and thus advantages reported in performance and efficiency when supplementing chopped forages to calves are not an artefact due to gut fill. Interestingly (and contrary to what could be expected a priori), provision of chopped oat straw to calves improved rumen passage rate of digesta and tended to improve ADG over time, without incurring increases in gut fill (in fact, gut fill was reduced by feeding oat straw) when compared with calves that were fed a pelleted starter (Castells *et al.*, 2013). The increase in passage rate and decreased gut fill can be explained mainly by a substantial increase (about 23%) in total dry matter intake compared with calves fed a pelleted starter feed alone (Castells *et al.*, 2012). In the same study, it was also reported that forage provision to calves increased almost four-fold the number of volatile fatty acid transporters in the rumen, a condition that should minimize rumen acidosis by actively removing acid from the rumen fluid.

Finally, depriving calves of forage during the pre-weaning phase may offer yet another physiological and dietary adaptation challenge to young calves during the transition when presented with forage for the first time. For example, Phillips (2004) reported that calves fed fresh grass during the milk-feeding period spent more time eating on pasture compared with those that received no forage before weaning.

Transitioning successfully

High intake of starter before weaning helps to ensure adequate intake and sustain a desirable growth rate after weaning (Kertz *et al.*, 1979). Data from 12 studies were adjusted for the random effect of study and a mixed-effects linear regression was performed between the study-adjusted ADG the week after weaning and starter intake the week before weaning. In the field, it is commonly recommended to wean calves when they consume about 1 kg/d of starter for three consecutive days. However, if an ADG of about 1 kg/d is sought around weaning time, calves should not be weaned until they consume at least 1.5 kg of dry feed (Figure 2). Weaning with intakes below 1.5 kg/d is possible, but growth, and potentially health, will be compromised.

With a proper nutritional scheme, transition calves (from a few days before to a few weeks after weaning) can grow approximately 1.2-1.3 kg/d at approximately 40% feed efficiency, resulting in the most profitable development stage that calves or heifers will undergo during their entire growing period. After weaning, it is recommended to continue transition with the same starter and chopped forage the animals were weaned on, and then change them to a ration that will progressively increase the proportion of fibre through inclusion of forage, starting with about 50 g/kg and finishing by the age of 4 months with a forage inclusion level of 150-200 g/kg. Forage inclusion increments should be performed weekly or fortnightly. The amount of energy and CP during this phase should be about 11.43 MJ/kg of ME and 170 g of CP/kg.

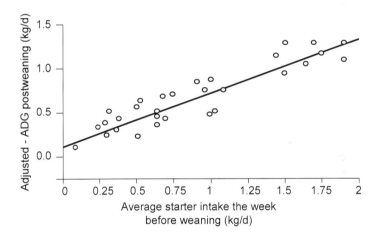

Figure 2. Linear relationship between daily starter intake the week before weaning and study-adjusted ADG the week after weaning of calves from different studies: adjusted-ADG post-weaning = 0.115 + 0.615 daily starter intake before weaning; R^2=0.82; $P < 0.001$; n=30 from Anderson et al., 1987; Jaster et al., 1992; Quigley et al., 1994; Quigley et al., 1996; Chua et al., 2002; Jasper and Weary, 2002; Quigley et al., 2006; Terré et al., 2006a; Terré et al., 2006b; Terré et al., 2009; Sweeney et al., 2010; Castells et al., 2012.

Weaning has usually been associated with a moment of stress. To minimize stress around weaning, it is commonly recommended to keep calves individually housed for an additional 1 or 2 weeks following weaning. However, a study conducted at the University of Minnesota (Ziegler *et al.*, 2008) compared performance of calves that were weaned and immediately moved to groups of 10 animals with those weaned and kept in individual stalls for an additional 14 d. The study reported no difference in performance during the first 112 d following weaning. Similarly, a study (Bach *et al.*, 2010) involving 240 female calves assessed the impact of grouping animals before weaning on ADG and health. Half of the calves were moved at 49 d of age (when MR was reduced from 2 to 1 daily dose) to super-hutches holding 8 calves; and the other half remained individually housed for an additional week after reducing the MR from 2 to 1 daily dose. Calves grouped at 49 d of age had a greater ADG and BW at 56 d of age as a result of a greater total solid feed consumption compared with those grouped at 56 d of age (Figure 3). More relevant, the study showed that calves weaned in groups had a lower number of respiratory episodes than those weaned individually, which would indicate that the level of stress (and thus debilitation of the immune response) was reduced when calves were grouped. It is important to note that MR (or milk) should be offered in a trough (no nipples) to avoid inter-sucking while calves are group-housed. Other studies have also shown that calves that are in groups before weaning have an improved behavioural response and a better ability to adapt to new environments or mates (De Paula Vieira *et al.*, 2012).

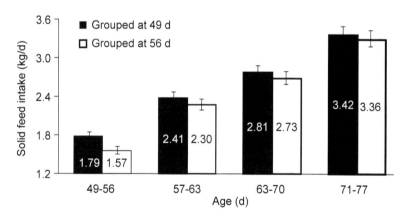

Figure 3. Solid feed intake of transition calves kept individually (for one additional week) or placed in groups of 8 animals at pre-weaning (49 d of age) time (Adapted from Bach *et al.*, 2010).

An important problem surrounding transition calves is bovine respiratory disease (BRD). Incidence of BRD has been reported to be directly related to group size of calves (Martin and Meek, 1986; Svensson *et al.*, 2003), and for this reason, it has been recommended to keep group size to about 6 to 10 animals (Svensson and Liberg, 2006; Bach and Ahedo, 2008). In addition, it has been reported (Bach *et al.*, 2010) that moving calves into groups at pre-weaning time (when MR allowance is decreased) improves calf performance and diminishes BRD incidence. In beef production systems, evidence exists that the health status and origin of calves being commingled seems to be important in determining BRD incidence (Step *et al.*, 2008), and, thus, grouping calves according to origin and BRD history may diminish morbidity after grouping. In fact, Bach *et al.* (2011) showed that that forming groups of animals with a BRD history should minimize the incidence of respiratory cases in those groups of calves formed by animals without a history of respiratory disease. Taking measures to minimize BRD incidence will not only have a short-term impact on growth and economic returns (i.e., less drug expenses), but will also have long-term return. Bach (2011) described a negative linear relationship between productive life and the number of BRD episodes that a cow experienced as a heifer (Figure 4).

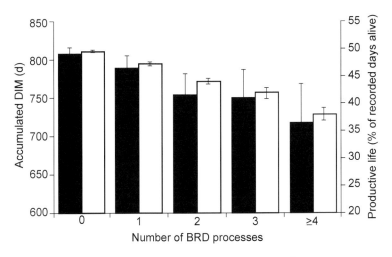

Figure 4. Accumulated productive life (days in milk (DIM); black bars) and productive life (as a percentage of productive days out of those recorded as alive; white bars) of cows as affected by the number of bovine respiratory disease (BRD) episodes experienced before first calving. Adapted from Bach (2011).

Nourishing and managing heifers

Once target age and BW at first calving have been set, the rate of growth at different stages of development should be defined. Assuming a calf is weaned at 63 d of age weighing 92 kg, for her to reach 650 kg (after calving) at 23 months of age she needs to grow at an average of 870 g/d. Because BW accretion is more efficient early in life than in later stages of growth, it makes economic sense to aim for fast growth rates before breeding. The recommendation is that heifers should be bred at 400 d of life (to achieve a first calving at 22-23 months) with an average BW of about 400 kg. Therefore, an optimum ADG between weaning (at 63 d of life) and breeding time (at 400 d) should be around 900 g/d. In the field, however, and also within some scientific schools, there is some generalized concern that growing excessively, above 700 g/d, during the pre-pubertal period might compromise mammary development and milking potential. This concern rises mainly from a study (Sejrsen et al., 1982) conducted in the early 1980s involving 10 heifers at two levels of nutrition during the pre-pubertal period and reported that heifers that grew at a rate of 1.3 kg/d had lower secretory cells (measured as DNA) than those that grew at a rate of 0.65 kg/d. However, age and BW were confounded in that study, with heifers growing at fast ADG being slaughtered at an early age. Daniels et al. (2009) evaluated the effect of ADG (ranging from 650 to 950 g/d) on mammary development and concluded that BW and age are the most important factors affecting mammary development, with rate of growth having a minimal impact. Furthermore, data gathered from more than 500 heifers (Bach and Ahedo, 2008), indicate that there is a weak, but positive, relationship between ADG between 66 and 400 d (breeding time) of life and future milk production during the first lactation. The relationship is weak (r = 0.21), but nevertheless it reinforces that rapid growth rates (up to 1.0 kg/d) achieved without inducing fattening the animals should not compromise future milk yield, and might actually increase milk yield.

To attain ADG of about 900 g/d, heifers during this period should consume TMR with 9.0 MJ of ME/kg and 150 g of CP/kg. It is important that the ratio between CP and ME is close to 7.0 to avoid fattening. Frequent checks of BW accretion are necessary to detect heifers that fall below targets. These heifers should be "delayed" or kept in the same pen where they were at the moment of BW check, remove the rest of heifers to the next age pen and bring younger and lighter heifers into that pen. Bach et al. (2006) showed that regrouping heifers that were growing below the average growth rate of their cohorts with a new set of younger and lighter animals resulted, in that study, in a dramatic increase in ADG during the following 2 weeks. After that time, "delayed" heifers could be moved into the next pen, as they would then continue to grow normally (Figure 5).

Feed costs represent the greatest expense associated with heifer rearing. Small improvements in feed conversion result in relative large savings. For this reason, it is important to monitor intakes continually and adjust the nutrient concentration of the ration to the maximum planned intake of the animals. For example, a diet with an energy concentration of 10.72 MJ of ME/kg formulated to provide 107.2 MJ of ME/d because the expected dry matter intake (DMI) is 10 kg/d could be reduced in cost per kilogram if actual DMI of the animals was 10.5 kg/d because energy concentration of the ration could then be reduced to 10.22 MJ of ME/kg to continue supplying the same energy level to the heifers. To apply this type of change

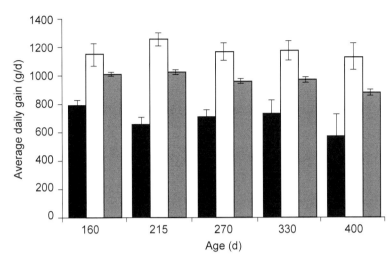

Figure 5. Average daily gain of non-delayed heifers (grey bars), and before (black bars) and after a regrouping (white bars) of delayed heifers. Error bars represent standard errors (Adapted from Bach *et al.*, 2006).

in the ration, feed intake should be monitored by recording daily offers and refusals. When such a feed monitoring system is implemented in conjunction with routine observation and weighing of heifers, it is possible to feed to attain maximum growth while minimizing feed costs without over-conditioning the animals.

In past years, there has been some emphasis on limit-feeding heifers to improve feed efficiency and avoid potential fattening. Hoffman *et al.* (2007) suggested that limit-feeding a diet with a nutrient concentration greater than normal (to ensure provision of all nutrients required) to raise heifers could be an alternative to control over-conditioning, and improve feed efficiency. In fact, Zanton and Heinrichs (2007) limit-fed young (130 kg BW) Holstein heifers for 35 weeks a diet containing 25% forage and compared these heifers with similar heifers receiving a greater allocation of a diet containing 75% forage. The authors reported no difference in ADG or skeletal growth between heifers in both groups. However, as nutrient concentration of a ration increases, cost per kilogram usually increases. Thus, a limit-feeding system is only economical if the increase in unit cost of the ration is offset by the expected decrease in DMI. Another concern with limit-feeding is that limit-feeding may potentially compromise future intake and thus milk yield. In the study of Zanton and Heinrichs (2007), future milk production did not differ between animals limit-fed at 5.3 kg/d (equivalent to 11% limit-fed) or controls fed at 5.9 kg/d. However, heifers of that age could be eating as much as 6.5 kg/d, and thus the "control" group was also "limit-fed" and more studies are needed that compare intakes around 6.5 kg /d with ≤ 6.0 kg/d.

Feeding the pregnant heifer

In contrast to observations that indicate that rapid growth rates during the pre-pubertal period are not detrimental (provided fattening does not occur), rapid ADG during pregnancy seems to be associated with impaired milk production. The metabolism of pregnant heifers is modulated by progesterone, which tends to foster fat disposition in preparation for lactation. Data collected from our research group indicate that rapid growth rates post-breeding are correlated with decreased milk performance for the first half of lactation (Bach and Ahedo, 2008). Similarly, Lascano *et al.* (2009) in a study with limit-fed heifers reported a tendency for decreased milk yield in heifers that grew at 1.1 kg/d compared with heifers that grew at 1.0 kg/d between about 360 d of age and calving. Thus, retarded growth resulting in below-target BW at breeding is difficult to correct because heifers will tend to use additional nutrients to gain condition (placing them at an increased risk of metabolic disorders after first calving). Therefore, nutrition until 400 d is crucial to ensure a successful rearing process. After conception, all that should be done is to ensure moderate growth and avoid over-condition. During the first months of pregnancy heifers should be fed rations providing 8.88 MJ of ME/kg and 160 of CP/kg.

Rations fed to heifers during the 2 months preceding calving should provide sufficient nutrients to ensure an ADG of 750 g/d. About 88% of this gain will be the result of foetal growth and its supporting structures (uterus, placenta, and fluids); the remaining 12% (about 100 g/d) corresponds to continued growth and development of the heifer. Most health problems in the high-producing dairy cow, of both metabolic and infectious nature, occur during early lactation and have been related to low energy intake and negative energy balance leading to ketosis and fatty liver as the two most common metabolic upsets. The majority of these health problems originate during the peri-parturient period. Traditionally, it has been recommended to feed high-energy rations during the pre-calving period to minimize body fat mobilization, ketosis, and fatty liver after calving and to adapt rumen microflora to high energy levels fed during lactation. In fact, NRC (2001) recommendations advocate a relatively high-energy ration (6.70 MJ of NEl/kg) before calving (with the intention of adapting the animal to a lactating ration and minimizing post-partum metabolic problems). Overfeeding heifers to the point that they become fat, however, can cause calving difficulties and metabolic problems postpartum. Furthermore, several studies (Rabelo *et al.*, 2003; Loor *et al.*, 2006) show that animals fed according to current NRC recommendations, allowing *ad libitum* access to high-energy diets during the dry period, show a greater decrease in feed intake before parturition and a lower feed intake postpartum; and several studies (Dann *et al.*, 2005; Douglas *et al.*, 2006; Loor *et al.*, 2006) suggest that heifers or cows that are moderately overfed during the dry period, even without becoming obese, may be placed at greater risk for peri-parturient health problems.

Thus, the currently recommended high energy content of the diet might actually be detrimental to the heifer. An average pre-partum heifer requires less than 96 MJ of ME per day, and feeding a ration containing 10.47 MJ/kg of ME would provide more than 108 MJ of ME per day. Therefore, it seems reasonable to feed pre-calving heifers rations containing about 8.8 MJ of ME/kg to supply their energy needs (96 MJ of ME/d). Regarding protein, rations during the pre-calving period of heifers should contain at least 140 g CP/kg DM to ensure sufficient metabolisable protein to sustain foetal growth as well as heifer development. Most or all the nutritional needs of pre-calving heifers can be achieved with high quality forage plus a small supplementation in the form of maize, maize gluten feed, soyabean hulls or barley, and a protein source such as soyabean meal or canola meal.

Conclusions

The way calves and heifers are reared will not only have an impact on the cost of rearing and health status and growth of calves and heifers, but will also have an impact on longevity and milking ability of these animals once they reach adulthood. Nutrient supply and hormonal signals at specific periods during development (both pre- and early post-natal) may exert permanent changes in metabolism, as well as changes in performance, body composition, and metabolic function of the offspring of livestock. Results from a meta-analysis concluded that about 225 kg of additional milk in the first lactation could be expected for each additional 100 g/d of growth during the first 2 months of life. However, calves fed high milk allowances tend to struggle during transition onto solid feed, and part of the growth advantage achieved before weaning may be lost due to (1) diminished consumption of nutrients, and (2) reduced digestibility. For this reason, fostering solid feed intake when providing large amounts of milk or milk replacer is imperative. Starter feed consumption can be improved by including 'palatable' ingredients in the formulation of the starter. Also, an effective method to foster solid feed intake of calves, contrary to what has been previously recommended, is to provide ad libitum access to poor quality (nutritionally) chopped straw or chopped grass hay. This practice has been shown to increase solid feed by 23% (and consequently growth also increases). Furthermore, forage provision to calves increased almost 4-fold the number of volatile fatty acid transporters in the rumen, a condition that should minimize rumen acidosis by actively removing acid from the rumen fluid. Growth accumulated during the pre-weaning period can be maintained by ensuring consumption of solid feed of at least about 1.5 kg of dry feed. An optimum ADG between weaning and breeding should be 900 g/d. Finally, rations fed to heifers during the 2 months preceding calving should provide sufficient nutrients to ensure an ADG of 750 g/d and it is recommended to keep pre-caving heifers on low-energy, high-fibre diets until calving.

References

Anderson, K.L., Nagaraja, T.G., Morrill, J.L., Avery, T.B. Galitzer, S.J. and Boyer. J.E. (1987) Ruminal microbial development in conventionally or early-weaned calves. *Journal of Animal Science,* **64**, 1215–1226.

Bach, A. (2011) Associations between several aspects of heifer development and dairy cow survivability to second lactation. *Journal of Dairy Science,* **94**, 1052–1057.

Bach, A. (2012) Ruminant Nutrition Symposium: Optimizing Performance of the Offspring: nourishing and managing the dam and postnatal calf for optimal lactation, reproduction, and immunity. *Journal of Animal Science,* **90**, 1835-1845.

Bach, A., Ahedo, J. and Ferrer, A. (2010) Optimizing weaning strategies of dairy replacement calves. *Journal of Dairy Science,* **93**, 413-419.

Bach, A. and Ahedo, J. (2008) Record keeping and economics for dairy heifers. (2008) *Veterinary Clinics of North America - Food Animal Practice.* **24**, 117-138.

Bach, A., Tejero, C. and Ahedo, J. (2011) Effects of group composition on the incidence of respiratory afflictions in group-housed calves after weaning. *Journal of Dairy Science,* **94**, 2001–2006.

Bach, A., Juaristi, J.L. and Ahedo, J. (2006) Case study: growth effects of regrouping dairy replacement heifers with lighter weight and younger animals. *The Professional Animal Scientist,* **22**, 358–361.

Bach, A., Domingo, L., Montoro, C. and Terré, M. (2013a) Short communication. *Journal of Dairy Science,* **96**, 4634–4637.

Bach, A., Terré, M. and Pinto, A. (2013b) Performance and health responses of dairy calves offered different milk replacer allowances. *Journal of Dairy Science,* **96**, 7790–7797.

Ballou, M.A. (2012) Immune responses of Holstein and Jersey calves during the preweaning and immediate postweaned periods when fed varying planes of milk replacer. *Journal of Dairy Science,* **95**, 7319–7330.

Barrier, A.C., Dwyer, C.M., Macrae, A.I. and Haskell, M.J. (2012) Short communication: Survival, growth to weaning, and subsequent fertility of live-born dairy heifers after a difficult birth. *Journal of Dairy Science,* **95**, 6750–6754.

Boland, T., Hayes, M.L., Sweeney, T., Callan, J.J., Baird, A.W., Keely, S. and Crosby, T.F. (2008) The effects of cobalt and iodine supplementation of the pregnant ewe diet on immunoglobulin G, vitamin E, T3 and T4 levels in the progeny. *Animal,* **2**, 197-206.

Castells L., Bach, A., Araujo, G., Montoro, C. and Terré, M. (2012) Effect of different forage sources on performance and feeding behavior of Holstein calves. *Journal of Dairy Science,* **95**:286–293.

Castells, L., Bach, A., Aris, A. and Terré, M. (2013) Effects of forage provision to young calves on rumen fermentation and development of the gastrointestinal tract. *Journal of Dairy Science,* **96**, 5226–5236.

Daniels, K.M., McGilliard, M.L., Meyer, M.J., Van Amburgh, M.E., Capuco, A.V. and Akers, R.M. (2009) Effects of body weight and nutrition on histological mammary development in Holstein heifers. *Journal of Dairy Science,* **92**, 499–505.

Dann, H.M., Morin, D.E., Bollero, G.A., Murphy, M.R. and Drackley, J.K. (2005) Prepartum intake, postpartum induction of ketosis, and periparturient disorders affect the metabolic status of dairy cows. *Journal of Dairy Science*, **88**, 3249–3264.

Davis Rincker, L.E., Weber Nielsen, M.S., Chapin, L.T., Liesman, J.S., Daniels, K.M., Akers, R.M. and VandeHaar, M.J. (2008) Effects of feeding prepubertal heifers a high-energy diet for three, six, or twelve weeks on mammary growth and composition. *Journal of Dairy Science*, **91**, 1926–1935.

De Paula Vieira, A., de Passillé, A.M. and Weary, D.M. (2012) Effects of the early social environment on behavioral responses of dairy calves to novel events. *Journal of Dairy Science*, **95**, 5149–5155.

DeNise S.K., Robison, J.D., Stott, G.H. and Armstrong, D.V. (1989) Effects of passive immunity on subsequent production in dairy heifers. *Journal of Dairy Science*, **72**, 552–554.

Douglas, G.N., Overton, T.R., Bateman, H.G., Dann, H.M. and Drackley, J.K. (2006) Prepartal plane of nutrition, regardless of dietary energy source, affects periparturient metabolism and dry matter intake in Holstein cows. *Journal of Dairy Science*, **89**, 2141–2157.

Drackley, J.K. (2008) Calf nutrition from birth to breeding. *Veterinary Clinics of North America - Food Animal Practice*. **24**, 55–86.

Faber S.N., Faber, N.E., McCauley, T.C. and Ax, R.L. (2005) Case study: effects of colostrum ingestion on lactational performance. *The Professional Animal Scientist*. **21**, 420-425.

Fall, C.H.D. (2011) Evidence for the intra-uterine programming of adiposity in later life. *Annals of Human Biology*, **38**, 410–428.

Heinrichs A.J. and Heinrichs, B.S. (2011) A prospective study of calf factors affecting first-lactation and lifetime milk production and age of cows when removed from the herd. *Journal of Dairy Science*, **94**, 336–341.

Hengst, B.A., Nemec, L.M., Rastani, R.R. and Gressley, T.F. (2012) Effect of conventional and intensified milk replacer feeding programs on performance, vaccination response, and neutrophil mRNA levels of Holstein calves. *Journal of Dairy Science,* **95**, 5182–5193.

Hill, T.M., Bateman, H.G., Aldrich, J. M.and Schlotterbeck, R. L. (2008) Effects of the amount of chopped hay or cottonseed hulls in a textured calf starter on young calf performance. *Journal of Dairy Science*, **91**, 2684–2693.

Hoffman, P.C., Simson, C.R. and Wattiaux, M. (2007) Limit feeding of gravid Holstein heifers: effect on growth, manure nutrient excretion, and subsequent early lactation performance. *Journal of Dairy Science*, **90**, 946–954.

Hough, R.L., McCarthy, F.D., Kent, H.D., Eversole, D.E. and Wahlberg, M.L. (1990) Influence of nutritional restriction during late gestation on production measures and passive immunity in beef cattle. *Journal of Animal Science*, **68**, 2622–2627.

Jahn, E., Chandler, P.T. and Polan, C.E. (1970) Effects of fiber and ratio of starch to sugar on performance of ruminating calves. *Journal of Dairy Science*, **53**, 466–474.

Jasper, J. and Weary, D.M. (2002) Effects of ad libitum milk intake on dairy calves. *Journal of Dairy Science*, **85**, 3054-3058.

Jaster, E.H., McCoy, G.C. Spanski, N. and Tomkins T. (1992) Effect of extra energy as fat or milk replacer solids in diets of young dairy calves on growth during cold weather. *Journal of Dairy Science*, **75**, 2524–2531.

Kertz, A.F., Prewitt, L.R. and Everett, J.P. (1979) An early weaning calf program: summarization and review. *Journal of Dairy Science*, **62**, 1835-1843.

Khan, M.A., Weary, D.M., Veira, D.M. and von Keyserlingk, M.A.G. (2012) Post-weaning performance of heifers provided hay during the milk feeding period. *Journal of Dairy Science*, **95**, 3970-3976.

Khan, M.A., Lee, H.J., Lee, W.S., Kim, H.S., Kim, S.B., Ki, K.S., Ha, J.K. Lee, H.G. and Choi, Y.J. (2007) Pre-and postweaning performance of Holstein female calves fed milk through step-down and conventional methods. *Journal of Dairy Science*, **90**, 876–885.

Kincaid, R. L. (1980) Alternative methods of feeding alfalfa to calves. *Journal of Dairy Science*, **63**, 91–94.

Lascano, G.J., Zanton, G.I., Suarez-Mena, F.X. and Heinrichs, A.J. (2009) Effect of limit feeding high- and low-concentrate diets with *Saccharomyces cerevisiae* on digestibility and on dairy heifer growth and first-lactation performance. *Journal of Dairy Science*, **92**, 5100–5110.

Loor, J.J., Dann, H.M., Guretzky, N.A.J., Everts, R.E., Oliveira, R., Green, C.A., Litherland, N.B., Rodriguez-Zas, S.L., Lewin, H.A. and Drackley, J.K. (2006) Plane of nutrition prepartum alters hepatic gene expression and function in dairy cows as assessed by longitudinal transcript and metabolic profiling. *Physiological Genomics*, **27**, 29–41.

Malmuthuge, N., Li, M., Goonewardene, L.A. Oba, M. and Guan, L.L. (2013) Effect of calf starter feeding on gut microbial diversity and expression of genes involved in host immune responses and tight junctions in dairy calves during weaning transition. *Journal of Dairy Science*, **96**, 3189–3200.

Margerison, J.K., Robarts, A.D.J. and Reynolds, G.W. (2013) The effect of increasing the nutrient and amino acid concentration of milk diets on dairy heifer individual feed intake, growth, development, and lactation performance. *Journal of Dairy Science*, **96**, 6539–6549.

Martin, S.W., and Meek, A.H. (1986) A path model of factors influencing morbidity and mortality in Ontario feedlot calves. *Canadian Journal of Veterinary Research*, **50**, 15–22.

McCance R.A. (1962) Food, growth, and time. *Lancet*, **2**, 671–676.

Miller-Cushon, E.K., C. Montoro, I.R. Ipharraguerre, and A. Bach. 2014. Dietary preference in dairy calves for feed ingredients high in energy and protein. Journal of Dairy Science, 97:1634–1644.

Montoro, C. E.K. Miller-Cushon, T.J. DeVries, and A. Bach. 2013. Effect of physical form of forage on performance, feeding behavior, and digestibility of Holstein calves. Journal of Dairy Science, 96:1117-1124.

NRC (2001) *Nutrient Requirements of Dairy Cattle*. National Academy Press, Washington, USA.

Obeidat, B.S., Cobb, C.J., Sellers, M.D., Pepper-Yowell, A.R., Earleywine, T.J. and Ballou, M.A. (2013) Plane of nutrition during the preweaning period but not the grower phase influences the neutrophil activity of Holstein calves. *Journal of Dairy Science*, **96**, 7155–7166.

Phillips, C.J.C. (2004) The effects of forage provision and group size on the behavior of calves. *Journal of Dairy Science*, **87**, 1380–1388.

Quigley, J.D., Wolfe, T.A. and Elsasser, T.H. (2006) Effects of additional milk replacer feeding on calf health, growth, and selected blood metabolites in calves. *Journal of Dairy Science,* **89**, 207–216.

Rabelo, E., Rezende, R.L., Bertics, S.J. and Grummer, R.R. 2003. Effects of pre- and postfresh transition diets varying in dietary energy density on metabolic status of periparturient dairy cows. *Journal of Dairy Science,* **88**, 4375–4383.

Roth, B.A., Keil, N.M., Gygax, L. and Hillmann E. (2009) Influence of weaning method on health status and rumen development in dairy calves. *Journal of Dairy Science,* **92**, 645–656.

Sejrsen, K., Huber, J.T., Tucker, H.A. and Akers, R.M. (1982) Influence of nutrition of mammary development in pre- and postpubertal heifers. *Journal of Dairy Science,* **65**, 793–800.

Step, D. L., Krehbiel, C.R., DePra, H.A., Cranston, J.J., Fulton, R.W. Kirkpatrick, J.G., Gill, D.R., Payton, M.E. Montelongo, M.A. and Confer, A.W. (2008) Effects of commingling beef calves from different sources and weaning protocols during a forty-two-day receiving period on performance and bovine respiratory disease. *Journal of Animal Science,* **86**, 3146–3158.

Stobo, I.J.F., Roy, J.H.B. and Gaston, H. J. (1966) Rumen development in the calf. 1. The effect of diets containing different proportions of concentrates to hay on rumen development. *British Journal of Nutrition,* **20**, 171–188.

Strozinski, L.L. and Chandler, P.T. (1971) Effects of dietary fiber and acid-detergent lignin on body fill of ruminating calves. *Journal of Dairy Science,* **54**, 1491–1495.

Suárez, B.J., Van Reenen, C.G., Stockhofe, N., Dijkstra, J. and Gerrits, W.J.J. (2007) Effect of roughage source and roughage to concentrate ratio on animal performance and rumen development in veal calves. *Journal of Dairy Science,* **90**, 2390–2403.

Svensson, C. and P. Liberg, P. (2006) The effect of group size on health and growth rate of Swedish dairy calves housed in pens with automatic milk-feeders. *Preventive Veterinary Medicine,* **73**, 43–53.

Svensson, C., Lundborg, K., Emanuelson, U. and Olsson, S.O. (2003) Morbidity in Swedish dairy calves from birth to 90 days of age and individual calf-level risk factors for infectious diseases. *Preventive Veterinary Medicine,* **58**, 179–197.

Sweeney, B.C., Rushen, J., Weary, D.M. and de Passillé, A.M. (2010) Duration of weaning, starter intake, and weight gain of dairy calves fed large amounts of milk. *Journal of Dairy Science,* **93**, 148–152.

Terré, M., Bach, A. and Devant, M. (2006a) Performance and behaviour of calves reared in groups or individually following an enhanced-growth feeding programme. *Journal of Dairy Research,* **73**, 480-486.

Terré, M., Tejero, C. and Bach, A. (2009) Long-term effects on heifer performance of an enhanced-growth feeding programme applied during the preweaning period. *Journal of Dairy Research,* **76**, 331-339.

Terré, M., Devant, M. and Bach, A. (2007) Effect of level of milk replacer fed to Holstein calves on performance during the preweaning period and starter digestibility at weaning. *Livestock Science,* **110**, 82-88.

Terré, M., Devant, M. and Bach, A. (2006b). Performance and nitrogen metabolism of calves fed conventionally or following an enhanced-growth feeding program during the preweaning period. *Livestock Science*, **105**, 109–119.

Thomas, D.B. and Hinks, C.E. (1982) The effect of changing the physical form of roughage on the performance of the early-weaned calf. *Animal Production*, **35**, 375-384.

Warner, R.G., Porter, J.C. and Slack, T. S. (1973) Calf starter formulation for neonatal calves fed no hay. Pages 116-122 in *Proceedings of the Cornell Nutrition Conference*. Cornell University, Ithaca, NY.

Wu G. 2006. Intrauterine growth retardation: Implications for the animal sciences. *Journal of Animal Science*, **84**, 2316–2337.

Zanton, G.I. and Heinrichs, A.J. (2007) The effects of controlled feeding of a high-forage or high-concentrate ration on heifer growth and first-lactation milk production. *Journal of Dairy Science*, **90**, 3388–3396.

Ziegler, D., Ziegler, B., Raeth-Knight, M., Larson, R., Golombeski, G., Linn, J. and Chester-Jones, H. (2008) Performance of post weaned Holstein heifer calves transitioned to group housing using different management strategies while fed a common diet. *Journal of Dairy Science*, **86**, 465 (Abstr.)

7

Recent Developments in Feed Enzyme Technology

H.V. MASEY O'NEILL, M.R. BEDFORD AND N. WALKER

AB Vista Feed Ingredients, Marlborough Business Park, Marlborough, Wiltshire, SN8 4AN

Introduction

Over the last twenty years feed enzyme use has developed far beyond the use of carbohydrases to combat viscosity. More targeted application is now possible with a better understanding of mechanisms both in degrading phytate and non-starch polysaccharides (NSP). This is invaluable when applying enzymes in diets containing novel ingredients and has dramatically increased the potential return on investment. It has also allowed the recent development of the use of NSP enzymes in high-fibre ruminant diets.

Advances in the use of phytase for non-ruminants

Many hundreds of trials show the efficacy of various phytase products at standard doses in releasing phosphorus and allowing reduction of inorganic phosphorous in non-ruminant diets. Certainly the long held understanding is that of phosphate release from the plant storage form of phosphorous, phytate. In more recent years, the concept of superdoses of phytase has arisen. This involves the consideration of phytate not only as a source of phosphorus, but also as an anti-nutrient. In this regard the target is almost complete de-phytinisation of the diet (as opposed to 50-70% destruction, which is the outcome with standard usage). In cereals such as wheat and maize, phytate is likely to be present at around 0.7%, and in by-products such as rice bran, as much as 5% (Selle *et al.*, 2007). Phytate, or IP-6, is considered an anti-nutrient as it interferes with gastric protein digestion through co-ordination with both pepsin and dietary proteins and thus provokes a compensatory increase in HCl and pepsin. This is not only a loss of potential net energy of gain but irritates the stomach and stimulates additional secretion of protective mucin and therefore increases endogenous loss. Phytate also sequesters valuable nutrients such as minerals, which are then excreted.

As phytate is converted to various lower phosphase esters by sequential removal of phosphate groups, the anti-nutritional effect is reduced, but recent evidence suggests that many phytases, particularly when used at a standard dose, struggle to convert IP4 to IP3 and as a result IP4 accumulates, particularly in the small intestine (Pontopiddan, 2012). This phosphoester is still very effective in precipitating Zn at ph5 and above and as a result can interfere with small intestinal digestion of protein as many intestinal proteases are Zn dependent. Finally, if phytate is completely dephosphorylated, the end product is inositol, which has been found in many studies to be a growth stimulant in broilers. For broilers and piglets, the performance improvement with a phytase superdose is likely to be as much as three to four points in feed conversion, as a result of IP6 and IP4 removal and provision of inositol. This is quite an advance in comparison to the usual matrix-driven approach where the target is to reduce cost (by removing added inorganic phosphate) and only maintain performance with the phytase. The most effective method for superdosing involves feeding sufficient phytase to release 85% of the phytate-P in the diet, which in most cases would result in use of a dose that would ordinarily release 0.2-0.22% phytate-P, with the application of a P matrix of no more than 0.15% phytate P. The reason for the apparent overfeeding of P is likely due to the provision of significant amounts of inositol, which may be phosphorylated post-absorption in order to perform some of its biological functions. Thus, ironically, superdosing may marginally increase the P requirements for maximal growth rate of non-ruminants.

Advances in understanding and application of NSP enzymes for non-ruminants

It is well understood that NSP enzymes improve performance by eliminating the nutrient-encapsulating effect of the cell wall and ameliorating viscosity problems particularly with arabinoxylans and mixed-linked β-glucans. Enzymes were found to have a positive effect on animal performance as long ago as the 1920s and the mechanism in barley-based diets was attributed to glucanases in the 1950s and 1960s (Fry *et al.*, 1958). Later, it was suggested that there is an accompanying benefit of liberating starch and proteins previously trapped within the cell wall (Hesselman & Aman, 1986). The identification of the true enzyme-substrate interaction lead to the realisation that the high arabinoxylan content in wheat and rye could be targeted with xylanases, which were shown to improve performance via the same mechanisms as β-glucanase in barley (Bedford & Classen, 1992). Unlike wheat, barley and rye, maize is not considered viscous and does not exert particularly high or troublesome gut viscosity. However, NSP enzymes may result in large performance benefits in diets containing maize (Masey O'Neill *et al.*, 2014) and low viscosity wheat (Persia *et al.* 2002).

Murphy *et al.* (2005) and others have shown that xylanase can improve gastric digestion of nutrients and used microscopy to visualise the breakdown of cell wall material, *in vivo*, with the use on an enzyme (Le *et al.*, 2013). It is suggested that the enzyme works directly to degrade the cell wall, releasing the contents for digestion by the animal. However, scanning electron micrographs taken during work by the authors (Masey O'Neill *et al.*, 2014) clearly shows the release of starch granules from the surface of maize particles but only little evidence of systematic breakdown of endosperm cell wall material with the use of a xylanase in an *in vitro* system (Figure 1). It appears that the enzyme has been more effective in de-anchoring starch from the cell wall material than breaking down cell wall material per se. This is a novel finding in that it suggests that there may be some xylan component involved in holding starch granules in place within an endosperm cell. Thus it appears the 'de-caging effect' is unlikely to explain the mode of action fully, particularly since the gastric phase conditions, particularly pH, limit the ability of the enzyme to act directly.

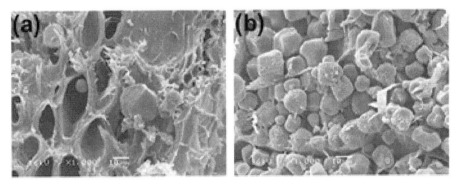

Figure 1. Ground maize incubated with a solution including (a) or excluding (b) xylanase (Econase XT, AB Vista Feed Ingredients, Marlborough, Wiltshire, UK). Reproduced from Masey O'Neill *et al.*, 2014

Following a large body of work in allied industries, the breakdown products of NSP enzymes are quite clear and can be identified. Accepting that the de-caging and viscosity reduction effects cannot alone explain the effects of NSP enzymes, it is suggested that there may be a prebiotic route by which the *products* of NSP enzyme degradation may themselves exert a beneficial effect. Courtin *et al.* (2008) showed that feeding wheat bran xylo-oligosaccharides, derived *in vitro* using a xylanase, to broilers resulted in the same performance effect as feeding a xylanase directly. Furthermore, in various species the fermentation of such fibre may exert systemic, hormonal effects on the gastric phase. For example, Goodlad *et al.* (1987) suggested that increased colonic fermentation in rats induced the release of Peptide YY (PYY), which leads to increased gastric retention time. Presumably, this leads to increased gastric digestion of nutrients such as protein, not only through longer exposure to pepsin but also the grinding action of the gizzard in poultry. It is interesting that amino acid digestibility studies note a consistent 15% reduction in the undigested fraction of all amino acids with enzyme addition, not just those concentrated in the cereal part of the ration, which further supports the hypothesis of an improvement in digestibility of the diet as a whole rather than only that of the cereal. Release of PYY in response to xylanase has been shown in initial experiments with broilers (Singh *et al.*, 2012).

It is possible that provision of too many or the wrong type of oligosaccharides early in the life of an animal may have detrimental effects on micro-flora but that eventually, as the population stabilises, provision of oligosaccharides may become beneficial. If this prebiotic mechanism is real, then the effect will not be limited to viscous cereal based diets but wherever there is substrate able to be enzymatically converted to oligosaccharides. For example, maize, like wheat, contains appreciable amounts of arabinoxylan which could be converted *in vivo* to arabinoxylo-oligosaccharide (AXOS) using a xylanase. However, enzyme dose and delivery are of critical importance as some oligosaccharides may be detrimental to performance. It is also important to consider where production of oligosaccharides may be limited. For example, it is conceivable that the xylan of highly processed products such as DDGS is so dramatically changed during processing that it is no longer prebiotic. It is also known that the longer material is exposed to enzyme, the smaller the fragments produced (Damen *et al.*, 2012). This could mean that xylan material which is already partially degraded may have all its beneficial effect removed by adding a further enzyme. It is difficult to assess the benefit of these prebiotic fragments from the literature as many fundamental methodologies regarding NSP involve analysis of component sugars, which does not elucidate the chain length or structure of the material. There is an argument for greater development in the understanding of oligosaccharides produced *in vivo* by enzyme action in production animals.

Advances in the use of exogenous fibrolytic enzymes (EFEs) in ruminant feeds

Although fibre-degrading enzymes (NSPases) and phytases are widely accepted and used commercially in the monogastric industry, only limited use has been made of exogenous fibrolytic enzymes (EFEs) for ruminants. This is perhaps due to the fact that, compared to the monogastric animal, the ruminant is regarded as being relatively efficient in terms of its ability to break down both fibre and phytate, and converts fibrous plant material into meat and milk by virtue of the complex microbial ecosystem residing in the rumen. A range of bacteria, anaerobic fungi and protozoa work together in a synergistic manner to help break down plant material, converting it into energy sources for the host. However, even though the ruminant is more efficient than a monogastric animal at breaking down plant cell walls, it has been estimated that plant cell wall digestibility in the total tract of ruminants is still less than 65% (Van Soest, 1994). Forages can make up a large proportion of the ruminant diet and can differ significantly in digestibility due to plant type and variety, with seasonal variation and growing conditions affecting degree of lignification and chemical composition. If the diet also contains a significant proportion of concentrate (>30%), Sub-Acute Ruminal Acidosis (SARA) may be induced, with rumen pH dropping below pH 5.8 for significant portions of the day. Below a rumen pH of 5.8, fibre digestion is impaired, due to the sensitivity of the fibrolytic microbial community to more acidotic conditions, leading to a reduction in both their numbers and enzymatic activity. In this instance, plant cell wall total tract digestibility may be reduced to as low as 50%, with only 30% occurring in the rumen (Beauchemin et al, 2001). Thus there is potential to improve fibre digestion, even in the ruminant animal.

In the late 1990s scientists investigated the potential of using EFEs derived from concentrated fungal fermentation extracts from Trichoderma as a means of further improving feed digestibility in the rumen and aiding fibre breakdown. These products were generally very high in xylanase and cellulase activity. Initial data was promising, with significant improvements in fibre digestion and animal performance being observed both in dairy and beef production systems. However, at that time, EFEs were not considered a commercially viable proposition due to the high costs of producing these EFEs relative to low feed prices and milk and meat price returns, and the technology was not adopted by the ruminant industry as quickly as it was by the monogastric industry. Today, with escalating feed costs combined with higher milk prices and better return on investments for dairy and beef, the potential use of EFEs in ruminant diets is being re-evaluated.

Potential mode of action of EFEs

Recent work using NIR has demonstrated that the predicted digestibility of a range of different forages could be significantly increased by spraying fungal fermentation extracts onto the surface of the fibre (Walker et al., unpublished data). Due to the high levels of hemicellulase and cellulase activity, the fibre starts to be pre-digested before the animal consumes it, as demonstrated by changes in NIR spectral analyses, leading to pre-digestion of the NDF and ADF component and increases in predicted D-value of up to 15% and predicted ME of up to 1.5 MJ/ kg DM. This has confirmed similar effects observed in some earlier studies where, after addition of EFEs to the forage, the concurrent reducing sugar release and change in NDF and ADF content was measured chemically (Hristov et al., 1996; Krause et al., 1998). It was hypothesised that this sugar release would act as a chemo-attractant for the rumen flora (Forsberg et al., 2000) and as a source of readily available carbohydrates, enabling rapid microbial growth, thus explaining the reduction in the lag time to digestion observed in several in situ studies. However, this sugar release would only represent a small portion of total carbohydrates potentially available and it is likely that several other factors are involved, leading to better feed digestibility. By action of the hemicellulose and cellulose degrading properties of the EFEs, pits are quickly formed in the surface of the fibre (McAllister *et al.*, 2001), leading to a roughened surface. When the treated forage is then consumed by the animal, this allows faster attachment and greater surface area colonisation by fibrolytic rumen microflora (Morgavi *et al.*, 2000). As a consequence, the lag time to digestion is decreased and overall DMd, NDFd and ADFd are increased, as demonstrated by both rumen in vitro and in situ measurements (Walker *et al.*, 2012; Holthausen *et al.*, 2011).

In a recent study (Holthausen *et al.*, 2011), daily treatment of a total mixed ration (TMR) for cows in early lactation with EFEs at two different dose rates led to a significant linear improvement in feed efficiency by up to 11%. This improvement in feed efficiency was driven lower dry matter intake coupled with no change in milk yield or component production. In a parallel side-study using fistulated animals fed the same diet and treated with the same product (Chung *et al.*, 2012), significant increases in the population sizes of fibre-digesting bacteria were observed, along with increases in *Ruminobacter amylophilus*, which is one of the first organisms to colonise grain in the rumen. The increase in the population size of this organism would imply better starch digestion could also be achieved, in addition to better fibre digestion and utilisation. The number of lactic-acid utilising bacteria, e.g. *Selenomonas ruminantium*, was also increased, and this is believed to occur due to the close relationship between this organism and one of the main fibre digesting bacteria, *Fibrobacter succinogenes*, which were also increased. Increased activity of *F. succinogenes*, which is a primary digester, releases more fermentation products which attract secondary digesters such as *S. ruminantium* and *R. amylophilus* to attach to and colonise feed particles (Cheng and McAllister., 1997). By increasing numbers of Selenomonads, rumen pH can be better regulated, further improving fibre digestion, and indeed no significant difference in rumen pH was observed between the control and treated groups in this study. This is perhaps surprising, as with greater fibre digestion, increased volatile fatty acid (VFA) production would be expected which could potentially cause a drop in rumen pH. This could be the case unless adequate rumen degradable protein is available in the diet to allow coupled fermentation and more microbial growth. In this study, although certain populations of micro-organisms were increased, the overall total number of bacteria, protozoa and anaerobic fungi were maintained. Instead, there was a shift in the microbial profile towards microbes which play a key role in breakdown of fibre and starch, indicating a better balanced fermentation. The change in the composition of rumen flora further confirms a potentially synergistic action between rumen flora and EFEs. This change towards more fibre digesting bacteria, coupled with the effects on the surface of the fibre, may explain some of the benefits in terms of better fibre and feed digestibility that have been observed in ruminant studies.

Potential benefits in dairy cow performance

A recent meta-analysis (Eun *et al.*, 2011) of 10 published studies demonstrated that using EFEs significantly increased DMI (+0.5kg/d, P=0.05) and milk yield (+2.3 kg/d, P<0.01), leading to significant improvements in feed efficiency (kg milk yield/kg DMI) from 1.52 to 1.59 (P= 0.01). Therefore, even though different dose rates and a range of diets were used, and fed to cows during the early stages of lactation, overall dairy cow performance was improved significantly. Commercial studies have also shown improvements in milk yield and components (N. Walker, personal observation). Generally milk production is increased on average in excess of 1 litre, with milk fat and milk protein also following suit, with more than 0.3% butterfat and 0.1% milk protein increases being observed. The increase in components generally reflects better rumen fermentation, with fibre utilisation driving acetate production, and better microbial protein yield driving increased milk protein. Measurements in the TMR and manure also confirm better fibre and starch digestion and feed utilisation between control and treated cows (R. Riewer, personal communication). However, effects are not always positive. In some studies, results have been inconclusive and no improvement in performance has been seen. These results seem to be driven by the composition of the EFEs used, the dose rate and the diet, interactions with the rumen flora and with the feed.

Potential benefits in beef performance

Although it would seem logical that the greatest effects of EFEs would be on dairy diets which contain a higher proportion of fibre, positive results have also been seen in beef production systems, both in the growing period and in the finishing period where the fibre content is lower. Beauchemin *et al.* (1999) showed that addition of EFEs to rolled barley grains, which comprised 90% of the diet fed to finishing cattle in a commercial feedlot, significantly increased live-weight gain (1.40 vs 1.53 kg/day, P<0.01) and numerically increased feed to gain by 10% (7.75 vs 6.92 kg DM/kg gain). Two recent studies (He *et al.*, 2014a, b) examined the effects on *in situ* feed digestibility of adding a similar EFEs mixture at two different levels to fistulated animals fed backgrounding and then intensive finishing diets. The backgrounding diet contained 50% barley silage, 25% barley, 15% wheat Dried Distillers Grains with Solubles (DDGS) and 10% hay; the finishing diet contained 60% rolled barley, 30% wheat DDGS and 10% barley silage. In the backgrounding diet, increasing the amount of EFE applied to the diet quadratically changed *in situ* DMd of wheat DDGS (61.1, 63.1 to 59.3%) and increased linearly *in situ* NDFd of barley silage

(14.9 to 18.9%). Crude protein digestion was also significantly increased in a linear manner. In the finishing diet, starch digestibility was significantly increased with increasing dosage treatment; however, no differences in digestibility of other nutrients were observed, nor were there any differences in ruminal pH or VFA production.

In conclusion, the potential benefits of using EFEs high in hemicellulase and cellulase activity in ruminant production are becoming obvious, especially as more data are collected. Further work is needed to understand the exact mechanisms involved, and perhaps why there is sometimes variability in responses. However, with the advent of low cost, consistent, high quality EFE products, and the need to improve feed digestibility, utilisation and efficiency, it is certain that more research efforts will be directed towards this interesting and new application.

References

Beauchemin, K. A., Rode, L. M. and Karren, D. (1999). Use of feed enzymes in feedlot finishing diets. *Canadian Journal Animal Science* 79, 243–246.

Beauchemin, K. A., Yang, W. Z. and Rode, L. M. (2001). Effects of barley grain processing on the site and extent of digestion of beef feedlot finishing diets. *Journal of Animal Science* **79**, 1925–1936.

Bedford, M.R. and Classen, H.L. (1992) *Journal of Nutrition*, **122**, 560-569.

Cheng, K.-J., and T. A. McAllister (1997) Compartmentation in the rumen. Pages 492–522 in *The Rumen Microbial Ecosystem*. P. N.Hobson and C. S. Stewart, ed. Blackie Academic & Professional, London, UK.

Chung Y.H., Zhou M., Holtshausen L., Alexander T.W., McAllister T.A., Guan L.L., Oba M. and Beauchemin K.A. (2012). *Journal of Dairy Science* **95**(3), 1419-1427.

Courtin C.M., Broekaert W.F., Swennen K., Lescroart O., Onagbesan O., Buyse J., Decuypere E., van de Wiele T., Marzorati M., Verstraete W., Huyghebaert G. and Delcour J.A. (2008). *Cereal Chemistry* **85**, 607-613.

Damen, B., A. Pollet, E. Dornez, W.F. Broekaert, I. Van Haesendonck, I. Trogh, F. Arnaut, J.A. Delcour and C.M. Courtin. (2012) *Food Chemistry* **131**, 111-118.

Eun, J.S., Williams, C.M. and Young, A.J. (2011). A meta-analysis on the effects of supplementing exogenous fibrolytic enzyme products in dairy diets on productive performance in early lactation. *Journal of Animal Science*. **89**, E-Suppl. 1/ *Journal of Dairy Science* **94**, E-Suppl. 1

Forsberg, C.W., Forano, E. and Chesson, A. (2000). Microbial adherence to the plant cell wall and enzymatic hydrolysis. P 79–97 *in* P. B. Cronje, ed. *Ruminant Physiology, Digestion, Metabolism, Growth and Reproduction*. CABI Publishing, Wallingford, UK.

Fry, R.E., J.B. Allred, L.S. Jensen and McGinnis. (1958) *Poultry Science* **37**, 372-375.

Goodlad, R.A., Lenton, W., Ghatei, M.A., Adrian, T.E., Bloom, S.R. and Wright, N.A. (1987) *Gut*, **28**, 221-226

He, Z.X., Walker, N.D., McAllister, T.A. and Yang, W.Z. (2014a) Effect of wheat dried distillers grains with soubles inclusion and fibrolytic enzyme supplementation on ruminal fermentation and digestibility in beef heifers fed backgrounding diet (abstract submitted to ADSA 2014 meeting).

He, Z.X., He, M.L., Walker, N.D., McAllister, T.A. and Yang, W.Z. (2014b) Using a fibrolytic enzyme to barley-based finishing diets containing wheat dried distillers grains with soubles, ruminal fermentation, digestibility, and growth performance in feedlot steers (abstract submitted to ADSA 2014 meeting).

Hesselman, K. and P. Aman. (1986) *Animal Feed Science and Technology*, **15**, 83-93.

Holtshausen L., Chung Y.H., Gerardo-Cuervo H., Oba M. and Beauchemin K.A.(2011) Improved milk production efficiency in early lactation dairy cattle with dietary addition of a developmental fibrolytic enzyme additive. *Journal of Dairy Science* **94**(2), 899-907.

Hristov, A. N., Rode, L. M., Beauchemin, K. A. and Wuerfel, R. L. (1996). Effect of a commercial enzyme preparation on barley silage *in vitro* and *in sacco* dry matter degradability. *Proc., West. Section, Am. Soc. Anim. Sci.* **47**, 282–284.

Krause M., Beauchemin K.A., Rode L.M., Farr B.I. and Nørgaard P. (1998) Fibrolytic enzyme treatment of barley grain and source of forage in high-grain diets fed to growing cattle. *Journal of Animal Science* **76**(11), 2912-20.

Le, D.M., Fojan, P., Azem, E., Pettersson, D, Pederson, N.R. (2013) *Cereal Chemistry* **90**, 439-444

McAllister, T.A., Hristov, A.N., Beauchemin, K.A., Rode, L.M. and Cheng, K.J. (2001). Enzymes in ruminant diets. Pages 273–298 in *Enzymes in Farm Animal Nutrition*. M. R. Bedford, and G. G. Partridge, ed. CABI Publishing. Marlborough, Wiltshire, UK.

Masey O'Neill, H.V., Singh, M. and Cowieson, A.J. (2014) Effect of exogenous xylanase on performance, nutrient digestibility, volatile fatty acid production and digestive tract thermal profiles of broilers fed wheat or maize-based diets. *British Poultry Science* **55**, 351–359.

Masey O'Neill, H.V., Smith, J.A. and Bedford M.R. (2014) *Asian-Australasian Journal of Animal Science* **27**, 290-301

Morgavi, D. P., Nsereko, V. L., Rode, L. M., Beauchemin, K.A., McAllister, T. A. and Wang, Y. (2000). A *Trichoderma* feed enzyme preparation enhances adhesion of *Fibrobacter succinogenes* to complex substrates but not to pure cellulose. *Proc. of the XXV Conference on Rumen Function*, Chicago, IL. p. 33 (Abstr.)

Murphy, T.C., Bedford M.R. and McCracken, K.J. (2004) *British Poultry Science* **45** Suppl 1 Pages, S61-2

Persia, M.E., Dehority, B.A. & Lilburn. M.S. (2002) *Journal of Applied Poultry Research*. **11**, 134-145.

Pontoppidan, K., Glitsoe, V., Guggenbuhl, P., Quintana, A. P., Nunes, C. S., Pettersson, D., and Sandberg, A. S. (2012) In vitro and in vivo degradation of myo-inositol hexakisphosphate by a phytase from Citrobacter braakii. *Archives of Animal Nutrition* **66**, 431-44.

Selle, P. H. and V. Ravindran. (2007) Microbial phytase in poultry nutrition. *Animal Feed Science and Technology* **135**, 1-41.

Singh, A., Masey O'Neill, H.V., Ghosh, T.K., Bedford, M.R. & Haldar. S. (2012) *Animal Feed Science and Technology* **177**, 194-203.

Van Soest, P. J. (1994). *Nutritional Ecology of The Ruminant.* 2nd ed.Cornell University Press, Ithaca, NY, USA.

Walker, N.D., Graham, H. and Miller Webster T.K. (2012) Effect of exogenous fibrolytic enzymes on rumen fermentation and feed digestibility during rumen in vitro incubations. Abstract in *Proc INRA-Rowett Gut Microbiology Meeting* p 139.

8

Enabling the Exploitation of Insects as a Sustainable Source of Protein for Animal Feed and Human Nutrition

FITCHES, E.C[1]., KENIS, M[2]., CHARLTON, A.J[1]., BRUGGEMAN, G[3]., MUYS, B[4]., SMITH, R[5]., MELZER, G[6]., WAKEFIELD, M.E.[1]

[1] *The Food and Environment Research Agency, York, UK;* [2] *Cabi, Delémont, Switzerland;* [3] *Nutrition Sciences N.V., Drongen, Belgium;* [4] *University of Leuven, Leuven, Belgium;* [5] *Minerva Communications Ltd, Andover, UK;* [6] *Eutema, Vienna, Austria*

Introduction

A growing global population and a rise in per-capita meat consumption is placing increasing pressure on the need to increase production of protein from sustainable sources. World population is expected to reach 9.6 billion by 2050, whilst the demand for meat, driven by an emerging global middle class is projected to grow by 73% from the level in 2010 (FAO, 2011). Protein is an important component of animal feed. Currently more than 80% of protein sources required for livestock rearing in the EU, such as soya and fishmeal, are imported from non-EU countries. This is problematic, as it can lead to market fluctuations and price rises in final products. Sustainable production of these protein sources is also a matter of debate. The UK alone currently imports approximately 2.5 million tonnes of soya per year, the majority of which is destined for animal feed, principally for pigs and poultry. Insects offer a promising alternative to conventional protein sources for animal feed. PROteINSECT is an international and multidisciplinary EU funded project that aims to facilitate exploitation of insects as an alternative protein source for animal feed. Incorporation of insects into animal feed could help to reduce the dependency of the EU upon external protein sources to feed its livestock. However, there are several areas of research that need to be undertaken before use of insect protein can be achieved at commercial levels. In addition, changes to the legislation that regulates animal feed in the EU would be needed before insect protein in animal feed is permitted. The research undertaken within the PROteINSECT project will advance knowledge in these key areas.

PROteINSECT – the concept

The principal objective of the PROteINSECT project is to facilitate exploitation of insects as an alternative source of protein for animal and human nutrition. Fly species are the most extensively researched insects for mass production and utilisation as animal feed. They can utilise a wide range of organic waste substrates for development, and this offers potential for low economic and environmental costs. In addition to conversion of waste to valuable products, such as protein and oils, dipteran larvae can also reduce the mass of organic waste, by up to 60% in 10 days. The remaining substrate can be used for added value in a number of ways, for example as fertilizer or compost (Figure 1). The focus of the PROteINSECT project is incorporation of insect protein into animal feed and input to the human food chain via utilisation as a component of the feed. Therefore, insect species that have potential for direct consumption by humans, for example crickets and grasshoppers, are not included in this project. The project is focussing on five key areas to provide a comprehensive evaluation of insects as a source of protein for animal feed:

1. Development and optimisation of fly production methods for animal feed production in European and developing countries.

2. Determination of the safety and quality of insect protein.

3. Evaluation of crude and processed insect protein in fish and monogastric (poultry and pig) feeding trials; animals for which insects form a natural part of their diet.

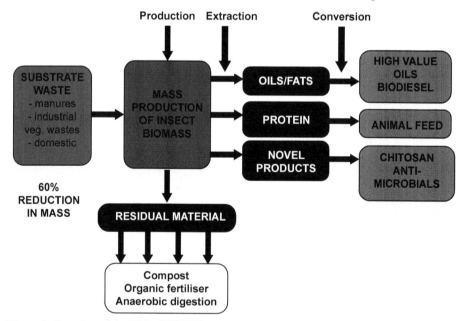

Figure 1. Overview of the PROteINSECT concept

4. Identifying environmental, social and economic life cycle impacts of insect-based animal feed production and use.

5. Building a pro-insect platform in Europe to encourage a holistic adoption of sustainable protein production technologies in order to reduce reliance of the feed industry on plant/fish derived proteins.

Insect production

Focus in PROteINSECT is placed on two fly species: the common housefly *Musca domestica* and the black soldier fly *Hermetia illuscens* (Figure 2), but other fly species are also being researched for their potential as a source of protein for animal feed.

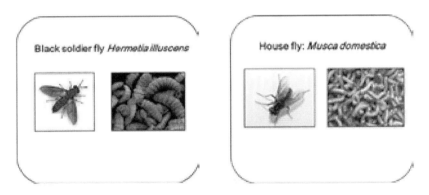

Figure 2. The black soldier fly, *Hermetia illuscens* and the house fly, *Musca domestica*

PROteINSECT has established new fly production systems in Europe, China and Africa, utilising animal manures and other organic waste materials (e.g. brewery waste, fish offal) as major substrates for larval growth (Figure 3a-c). A number of factors, including optimisation of rearing substrates, designs for collection and drying of larvae, determination of oviposition attractants and the control of natural enemies, are being investigated in order to improve production efficiency and potential for scale-up. Potential solutions to bottlenecks in rearing systems, such as maintenance of adult cultures and supply of eggs to maximise larval yields, are being explored. Variability of the substrate has also been shown to be a factor in optimising yield from various systems. In all systems larvae are harvested at the larval stage and supplied as crude dried insects for further studies, in particular to examine the nutritional profile and safety of the larvae.

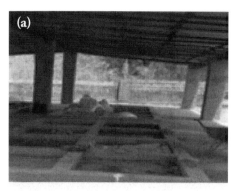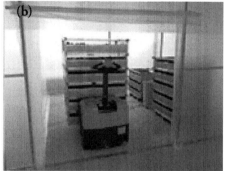

Figure 3. Production of *Musca domestica* in (a) Mali and (b) China

Quality and safety

Although the potential use of insects as a source of nutrition for domestic animals/fish has been recognised for several decades (e.g. Bondary and Sheppard, 1987; Newton et al., 2005; Hem et al., 2008), this has not yet led to any significant replacement of traditional plant/fish-based protein used for livestock production. This is largely due to systems being explored and developed on a local, isolated level with no integration or co-ordinated development of know-how to enable adoption at national and international levels. This is starting to change, however, and in the last couple of years companies have been set up to commercialise production of protein and other products from insects once legislation permits their use in animal feed. Such companies include Agriprotein (South Africa), Enterra (Canada), Protix Biosystems (The Netherlands) and YInsect (France).

A recent study comparing nutritive characteristics of a range of insects has shown that the amino acid profile of dipteran insects is superior to soybean meal and more similar to fishmeal (Barroso et al., 2014). Total protein and lipid contents of *M. domestica* larvae are widely reported to reach approximately 60% and 25% of dry weight respectively. Ongoing work in PROteINSECT is investigating the impact of rearing systems on these values, also considering the nutritional properties imparted by the amino and fatty acid profiles.

A major consideration in the use of any novel feed product is to demonstrate safety. The insect larvae themselves may present some hazards, for example allergens or anti-nutritional substances, but the substrates on which the insects are reared could also contain undesirable substances, particularly given that the larval rearing substrates are waste products (Figure 4). Little published data are available in relation to risks of using insects in feed and how these risks might be mitigated. Chemical safety testing in the PROteINSECT project will include analysis of heavy metals (e.g. cadmium, mercury, lead), pesticides (multi residue screen for a total of 416 compounds), dioxins

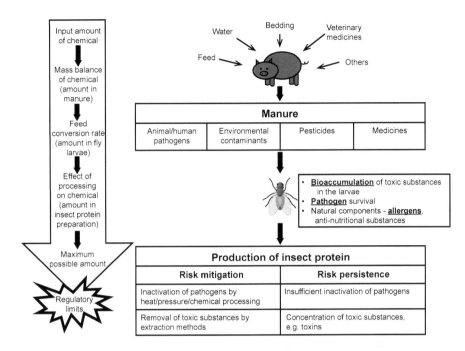

Figure 4. Potential for safety risks in the insect production chain

(17 compounds), polychlorinated biphenyls (PCBs) (25 compounds), polycyclic aromatic hydrocarbons (PAHs) (28 compounds), veterinary medicines (68 EU regulated compounds and a further 492 compounds including those known to be used worldwide) and mycotoxins. Microbiological risks, such as potential for persistence of *Salmonella* spp, *Campylobacter, Listeria monocytogenes* and Hepatitis E, will be evaluated. Initial studies on nine samples of larvae of different fly species using a recently developed and validated loop mediated isothermal amplification (LAMP) assay have all been shown to be negative for *Salmonella* species. Allergenicity is also a potential problem for insect protein. Allergenicity may occur in animals consuming feed in which insect protein is incorporated or in humans who subsequently consume fish or meat derived from these animals. There is little published information on insect allergens, but potentially allergenic proteins include tropomyosin. This is the main allergen found in shellfish and the protein sequence is similar to that found in insects. PROteINSECT will examine the potential for allergenicity of protein from larvae of the fly species used in the project. Downstream analysis of meat derived from insect reared animals will also be undertaken in relation to safety and quality (e.g. taints).

Much of the work to date on insect protein in animal feed has made little or no attempt to process the insect material produced. In PROteINSECT processing options for improving the nutritional status of insect protein are being investigated and nutritional analysis will provide key information enabling feed formulation and design of appropriate animal feeding trials. Where possible feeding trials will be conducted using both crude and refined material to enable the benefits of protein refining to be evaluated. Fish feeding trials will be carried out using representative species in China, Mali, Ghana (such as tilapia, *Oreochromis* sp.) and in the UK (Atlantic salmon, *Salmo salar*). Poultry are globally a major animal protein source and chicken feeding trials will be conducted in China, Mali and Belgium. Pigs constitute a major protein source for human consumption in Europe, and trials will be carried out in Belgium.

Possibilities for obtaining valuable by-products from insects, such as lipids, vitamins, minerals and chitin as well as fertilisers from the digested substrates, are also being considered. Lipids are a large component of the fly larvae. The crude fat content in meal produced from house fly larvae ranges from 140.8 to 272.9 g/kg (Fasakin *et al.*, 2003; Aniebo *et al.*, 2008, Pretorius, 2011), probably depending on the feed substrate for the larvae (Pretorius, 2011). The proportion of fat in *M. domestica* larvae can vary depending on age of the larvae and processing method used. In a study by Aniebo and Owen (2010), fat content increased from 224 to 273 g/kg on a dry matter basis as age of oven dried larvae increased from two to four days. The principal fatty acids found in *M. domestica* larvae and pupae are palmitic, palmitoleic, oleic and linoleic (St-Hilaire *et al.*, 2007; Hwangbo *et al.*, 2009). The potential to convert oils derived from the black soldier fly to biodiesel has been demonstrated (Li *et al.*, 2011a,b). Both *M. domestica* and *H. illucens* are sources of lipids that have a range of uses for nutrition and also with potential for exploitation as sustainable energy sources.

Life cycle analysis

Data obtained from insect production scenarios, quality and safety analysis, and feeding trials will form the basis for assessments of environmental, social and economic life cycle impacts of insect based animal feed production systems. The overall objective of this component of PROteINSECT is to facilitate design of optimised and sustainable production systems suitable for adoption by both small and large-scale operations in different geographical locations. Following a general life cycle assessment (LCA) framework, impacts (e.g. production efficiency, energy use, land use) will be quantified and compared to conventional feed assessments. Experimental data from feeding trials will be used to conduct assessments for fish, pigs and poultry that will be evaluated under different production scenarios. Ultimately LCA analyses will enable policy and technical recommendations to be provided for establishment of economically viable and efficient fly rearing systems in different locations.

Regulatory issues and consumer acceptance

Use of insects in animal feed is not currently recognised or specified in European legislation or regulation and this presents a major barrier to development of industrial insect-rearing plants. PROteINSECT is engaging with policy makers in order to support introduction of enabling legislation, and a recent report mapping current EU legislation has identified key challenges that need to be addressed (Smith and Pryor, 2013). These include authorisation of insect processed animal protein for use in non-ruminant feed, the need for solid scientific evidence of the safety of products to permit rearing of insects on animal manures, and legislation to address novel issues associated with mass production (Table 1). The regulations currently prohibit use of processed insects as a feed material, because the TSE regulation prohibits feeding of all farmed animals with processed animal protein (PAP), which includes protein derived from insects, except for PAP derived from non-ruminants (including insects) that may be fed to aquaculture species. However, the requirement for PAP to be processed in a registered slaughterhouse means that this is not technically possible. The substrate on which insects are reared is also a consideration. Insects produced for feed would be classed as "farmed animals", for which only category 3 material is allowed as a feed source. Manure is a category 2 material and therefore is not permitted to be fed to "farmed animals". Other issues such as the welfare of insects raised for use in animal feed will also need to be considered together with the health and welfare of those working in the industry.

Table 1. Regulations pertaining to the potential use of insect protein in animal feed

EC Regulation 178/2002	General principles and requirements of food law
EC Regulation 183/2005	Requirements for feed hygiene
EC Directive 2002/32	Undesirable substances in animal feed
EC Regulation 767/2009	Placing on the market and use of feed
EU Regulation 68/2013	Catalogue of feed materials
EC regulation 999/2001	Rules for the prevention, control and eradication of certain transmissible spongiform encephalopathies
EC Regulation 1069/2009	Laying down health rules as regards animal by-products and derived products not intended for human consumption
EC Regulation 56/2013	Amending Annexes I and IV to Regulation(EC) No 999/2001

Consumer acceptance is key to the successful commercial utilisation and adoption of insects as a source of protein for livestock. As such focus is also placed on activities such as monitoring relevant media coverage and gauging consumer attitudes. Coverage in world-wide media over the last 12 months has been considerable with the tone of such coverage overwhelmingly positive regarding use of insects in both feed and food. An initial consumer survey conducted in 2014 by PROteINSECT highlighted the need for more information to be made available (88.2% of 1302 respondents), but has suggested that the public are generally accepting of the use of insects in animal feed.

PROteINSECT is consulting with key stakeholder groups (e.g. producers of feed and feed ingredients, consumers, government) to generate a core 'business case' for use of insects in animal feed. Ultimately presentation of a White Paper to the European Parliament will ensure that regulatory aspects and consumer issues are brought to the political arena. Our aim is to build a pro-insect platform in Europe to encourage adoption of sustainable protein production technologies in order to alleviate reliance of the feed industry on plant/fish derived proteins.

Conclusion

There is clear potential for use of insects as a component of animal feed, together with the possibility to reduce waste volumes. There is also potential to improve land use efficiency as the land that would be needed to produce a given amount of insect protein from waste streams would be considerably less than that currently used to grow crops for inclusion as a protein source in animal feed. The economics of the process could be improved through production of other high value products such as lipids and chitin. However, further research is needed to ensure the safety of insect derived products and to maximise yield of insects, ideally through development of automated systems. Changes in legislation would also be needed.

Acknowledgements

The research leading to these results has received funding from the European Union's Seventh Framework Programme for research, technological development and demonstration under grant agreement n° 312084

References

Aniebo, A.O. and Owen, O.J. (2010). Effects of age and method of drying on proximate composition of housefly larvae (*Musca domestica*) meal (HFLM). *Pakistan Journal of Nutrition*, 9(5), 485-487.

Aniebo, A.O. Erondu. E.S. and Owen, O.J. (2008). *Proximate composition of housefly larvae (Musca domestica) meal generated from mixture of cattle blood and wheat bran*. Department of Animal Science and Fisheries, University of Port Harcourt, Nigeria.

Barroso, F.G., de Haro, C., Sánchez-Muros, M.J., Venegas, E., Martiez-Sánchez, A. and Pérez-Bañón, C. (2014). The potential of various insect species for use as food for fish. *Aquaculture*, 422-423, 193-201.

Bondari, K. and Sheppard D.C.(1987). Soldier fly, *Hermetia illuscens* L., larvae as feed for channel catfish, *Ictalurus punctatus* (Rafinesque), and blue tilapia, *Oreochromis aurues* (Steindachner). *Aquaculture and Fisheries Management*, 18, 209-220.

FAO. (2011). *World livestock 2011 – livestock in food security.* FAO, Rome.

Fasakin, E.A., Balogun, A.M. and Ajayi, O.O. (2003). Evaluation of full-fat and defatted maggot meals in the feeding of clariid catfish, *Clarias gariepinus*, fingerlings. *Aquaculture Research* 34(9), 733-738.

Hem, S., Toure, S., Sagbla, C. and Legrande, M. (2008). Bioconversion of palm kernel meal for aquaculture: experiences from the forest region (Republic of Guinea). *African Journal of Biotechnology* 7, 1192-1198.

Hwangbo, J., Hong, E.C., Jang, A., Kang, H.K. Oh, J.S., Kim, B.W. and Park, B.S. (2009). Utilization of house fly maggots, a feed supplement in the production of broiler chickens. *Journal of Environmental Biology*, 30(4): 609-614.

Li, Q., Zheng, L., Cai, H., Garza, E., Yu, Z. and Zhou, S. (2011a) From organic waste to biodiesel: black soldier fly, *Hermetia illucens*, makes it feasible. *Fuel*, 90:1545-1548.

Li. Q., Zheng, L., Qiu, N., Cai, H., Tomberlin, J.K. and Yu, Z. (2011b). Bioconversion of dairy manure by black soldier fly (Diptera: Stratiomyidae) for biodiesel and sugar production. *Waste Management*, 31:1316-1320.

Newton, L et al. (2005) Unpublished report http://www.cals.ncsu.edu/waste_mgt/smithfield_projects/phase2report05/cd,web%20files/A2.pdf

Pretorius, Q. (2011). The evaluation of larvae of *Musca domestica* (common house fly) as protein source for broiler production. MSc thesis Stellenbosch University.

Smith, R. and Pryor, R. (2013). Mapping exercise report with regard to current legislation and regulation: Europe and Africa & China. Available at www.proteinsect.eu.

St-Hilaire, S., Sheppard, C., Tomberlin, J.K., Irving, S., Newton, L., McGuire, M.A., Mosley, E.E., Hardy, R.W. and Sealey, W. (2007). Fly pre-pupae as a feedstuff for rainbow trout, *Oncorhynchus mykiss*. *Journal of the World Aquaculture Society*, 38(1): 59-67.

9

Using Animal-Oriented Indicators and Benchmarking for Continuously Improving Animal Health and Welfare

THOMAS BLAHA

University of Veterinary Medicine Hannover, Field Station for Epidemiology, Buescheler Str. 9, D-49456 Bakum, Germany

Societal changes

The intensification of agriculture as basis for feeding the human population has been regarded as progress for centuries, since the fewer people of a population are needed to produce the necessary food for all people, the more human resources are available for industrial and cultural progress. This platitude has been true as long as the food supply has been staying behind the demand for plenty and high-quality food for everybody, but this societal consensus is almost abruptly changing, when there is an oversupply of food, even if this is only perceived by the affluent parts of the population in question: agriculture, and especially producing food from and with animals is increasingly questioned and criticized.

This very rough pattern of agricultural development and the change of its societal acceptance can be exemplified by the relatively short period from World War II until today. Regarding the area of agriculture and food supply, three phases of the post-war development can be differentiated: "Shortage", "Risks" and "Guilt".

Shortage: During the war and particularly afterwards, the shortage of food was ubiquitous and agriculture was almost everywhere characterized by a small-scale structure. The need for food was enormous and aggravated by the growing urbanization and industrialization that started in the 1950s. In the "West", farmers benefited from the demand and a process of "growing or vanishing" started the intensification of agriculture: efficient farms grew, less efficient farms died away. In the "East", totalitarian regimes decided to become politically and economically independent of the "West", which resulted in an agricultural development that was designed to guarantee self-sufficiency, at least in the area of food. The Eastern communistic states developed in the early 1970s huge agriculturally used fields for crop production and likewise huge units for food animals (e.g. in East Germany sow units up to 5,000 sows and dairy farms up to 18,000 milking cows. These units became a kind of blueprint for highly intensive and efficient large-scale animal production, which is common in many industrialized countries. The major characteristic of this "shortage" phase was (on either side of the "iron curtain") that there was a non-debated consensus about the urgently needed intensification of agriculture. The goal was "never ever hunger again", and "plenty of affordable food for everybody". Publicly funded research contributed to technical developments that helped considerably to reduce labour needed per food entity. Many of the developments criticized nowadays, such as cages for laying hens, were greatly appreciated as efficiency and hygiene improvements of egg production. Improvement of productivity was the mantra of this period with almost full societal consensus.

Risks: There were two major and unrelated developments that started the growing questioning "Is everything right what we have done so far?", which is on the one hand the thought provoking first report of the "Club of Rome" warning that intensification, having negative side effects, may have gone too far, and on the other the emergence of Bovine Spongiform Encephalitis (BSE) in cows, reminding society that not only plenty of food for all is important, but also the safety of all products for human consumption. The demand for an "end of growth" and the initially not understood BSE raised a lot of questions and triggered the feeling that we need a change in our understanding and our procedures in the area of food production and consumption. Whereas the demand for a "zero-growth" stayed almost unheard, the occurrence of BSE and the simultaneously steeply increase of infections in humans by Salmonella (S.) Enteritidis stemming from eggs and chicken meat was seen as a major crisis. This crisis resulted in a deep distrust in the safety of our food, and in a quite drastic paradigm shift in the European approach to guarantee that our food is fit for human consumption. The European Regulation (EC) 178/2002 (the so-called mother regulation for the new European food safety legislation) turned the traditional mostly end product oriented inspection of food into a food chain oriented process improvement, with HACCP principles and information exchange up and down the food chain being the major elements of this new strategy. Managing the risks rather than managing the crises became the new mantra in this period. In hindsight, it must be admitted that the food safety risks that triggered the paradigm shift (zoonotic pathogens, residues such as dioxin and other chemical substances) were soon under control, but still the distrust is deeply rooted in most European populations: although we now have food that has never been as safe as today, the perception is that with the increasing industrialization of food production (preservatives, food additives, pesticide and herbicide use in crop production and the use of antibiotics in food animals), the food that is not "natural" or "organic" is health threatening and unsafe. However, although there is a kind of "bio-hype" and the demand for organic food is slightly increasing, the majority of the European population is still buying conventional food, especially in the case of meat.

Guilt: Beginning in the late 1990s, the attitude of the general society and consumers, propelled by activist groups, moved first slowly, but soon more and more rapidly towards criticism of what is done in the agricultural and food sector. Especially meat production and thus meat consumption is blamed for two major negative consequences of the intensive agriculture and an abundant supply of high-quality food rich in animal protein: the controversially discussed climate change and the "cruelty to animals due to factory farming". Vegetarianism and veganism are justified more and more by moral considerations that people do not have the right to kill animals, and if at all, at least the animals should be raised and cared for in small-scale family farming settings. This development is based on a quite radical change in societal attitude towards animals in general and a change in the way people interpret and value the human-animal bond. Animals are seen as living creatures with an intrinsic value that gives animals their own dignity. This is mainly promoted by urban citizens who live with pet animals that are increasingly often companions that have the same status as family members and friends. The latter is definitively not the only driver of the changes in the human-animal relationship, but one of the stronger determinants of the described changes in attitude. Other drivers are such as:

- the complete lack of knowledge about hunger and food shortage in the younger generation,

- a growing detachment of the urban population from any knowledge about and experience with agricultural processes as the major basis of our food supply,

- the lack of understanding that the currently low food prices in most European countries, which most people enjoy, cause farmers to constantly look for ways to reduce costs, and that, if they invested a considerable amount of money into better conditions for their animals, the market would not take their products at the prices the farmers would need to get their costs back – retailers would simply switch to cheaper products such as imports from low-cost countries,

- the bad feeling with wrong-doing by living in "unlimited" luxury, and

- the good feeling with being able to stigmatize certain professional groups and, thus, to blame others (e.g. farmers) for the perceived wrong-doing.

All in all this period is characterized by the fact that especially activist groups demand more and more animal welfare and organic or more natural production systems (e.g. free-range and out-door husbandry). Consumption of food is still oriented towards "cheap" food, however, and pricing in the retail sector is supporting this by offering especially meat products at extremely low prices to lure consumers into buying those groceries where all other products are then expected also to be as cheap as the advertised cheap meat. Another characteristic is that there are several misperceptions about animal production: e.g. it is simply not true that big animal units necessarily mean cruelty to animals and that small animal holdings mean always happy animals.

Why are we behind expectations?

The result of the development described above is that there is a widening gap between on the one hand what critical parts of the population and sophisticated well-to-do consumers expect regarding husbandry systems and handling of animals for food production and on the other how farmers (have to) raise and handle their animals. Traditionally, such situations call for new regulations and laws and/or for raising the minimal standards set by existing regulations and laws. National governments and more and more often also the EU have been trying to close or at least to narrow the gap. However, even in countries with very strict regulations, and which regularly come up with stricter regulations to guarantee a decent animal welfare standard, the gap remains more or less as wide as it was before raising the minimal standards.

Figure 1 illustrates this: the top line shows that the increase of societal expectations is a steady process, whereas the bottom line shows that the increase in legal minimal standards goes only upwards like a stair case, since it takes time and a lot of e.g. parliamentary discussions before an existing regulation is amended or a new law is issued. Moreover, the time lags between raised expectations and issuing new rules leads to the fact that even at the time a new regulation is issued, it does not satisfy everybody.

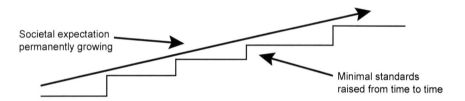

Figure 1. The varying gap between steadily increasing societal expectations and the "limping behind" of raising legal standards that can only take place in a "staircase" manner

This allows for the question whether raising the legal standards every now and then to "catch up" with the rising demands for welfare standards is the right or at least the only measure to meet the expectations of the welfare activist groups and the critical part of the general society. The answer is simply "No", for which there are four major reasons:

a) the objective to satisfy the expectations of animal welfare activists is a "moving target", since fulfilling the wishes of today produces new wishes for tomorrow,

b) raising legal standards, especially in democratic political systems, is not only time consuming, but is also a process for which consensuses must be found,

c) legal standards are nothing more than minimal requirements that naturally stay behind higher expectations and that most farmers only "gruntingly" comply without trying to do more, and

d) not all farmers adopt immediately higher standards and not every farmer complies with the new legal standards, which leads to the fact that there are always, in regard to animal health and welfare, well doing and poor doing farmers.

This means that closing the gap, or keeping it as narrow as critical people feel almost content with the conditions in which our food animals live, needs an additional process, which should be a systematic approach to implementing the principles of continuous improvement, which many other industries have already adopted.

How to manage continuous improvement?

One of the basic principles in the realm of quality assurance and quality management in any area of human activities is that "you can only improve what you measure". There are two groups that potentially try to use the principles of continuous improvement: a) single producers or clusters of producers that want to maintain their access to the market in a world of increasing quality demands, and producers or clusters of producers that want to create a niche for their products with high quality or unique specifications, and b) state authorities that are responsible for making sure that producers comply with the minimal standards set by legal regulations – they need measurements for assessing the degree of compliance to find out who is not only violating the current regulations, but nowadays also to recognize who has room for improvement to be asked to reduce the identified deficiencies in the care for their animals. The latter has become acutely important with putting the EU Regulation Reg. (EC) 178/2002 in force, which decidedly asks for applying measures of a risk-oriented control system, instead of random sample controls. The point of this is: state controls are to be concentrated more on those production sites that have either a history of non-compliance and/or are suspected of non-compliance since there are indications for that. If state authorities succeed in applying such risk-oriented controls, they will be able to demand improvements from those that need to do a better job, and they save time and labour by controlling those that can be trusted less often. The EU has issued a separate regulation (Reg. [EC] 882/2004), which applies to all kinds of state controls along the food chain (feed mill, food animal herds and flocks, abattoirs, processing plants and retail outlets).

The principles of risk-oriented controls are not too complicated to apply to feed mills, abattoirs, processing plants and retail outlets, since their number is so low that they all are relatively often controlled and built up quite rapidly a "control history", which makes risk-oriented controls feasible. However, the huge multitude (compared to feed mills, abattoirs etc.) of food animal farming units means much longer intervals between state controls of food animal herds and flocks to assure their compliance with legal standards. With increasing demands for better husbandry systems and a better care for the animals, and especially with each "scandal", there is an increasing perception that the state controls fail to identify shortcomings in applying state of the art procedures on too many farms. For too long, state controls have concentrated only on compliance of farms with the legal standards for housing conditions such as square metres per animal and measurements of slatted floors etc. (= husbandry-oriented indicators). This concentrating on so called input criteria totally overlooked the fact that animals, which are kept under housing condition that meet all minimal standards, but are poorly cared for, can suffer more than animals that are kept under sub-optimal housing conditions, but are excellently cared for.

Which animal-oriented indicators are useful?

Therefore, animal-oriented indicators per herd or flock such as frequency of disease, frequency of injuries, lameness, mastitis in cows, food lesions in poultry are needed to assess the quality of the animals' life and of the quality of the stockmanship and the empathy for animals of the animal caretakers.

The basic principle for any system that uses animal-oriented indicators for implementing continuous improvement processes to improve the animal health and welfare status of food animal herds and flocks are:

1. recording standardized findings related to animal health and welfare per animal population,

2. calculating a Herd-Health-Welfare-Index (HHWI), e.g. in points per criterion and sum the points up to an index, and

3. benchmarking those herds or flocks, the HHWI of which is calculated in the same manner.

Animal-oriented indicators can be recorded at farm level (e.g. mortality rate and antibiotic use expressed in days that animals of the herd or flock are treated with any antibiotic substance, which is expresses as Animal-Treatment-Index (ATI), and at abattoir level. The latter can and should be done at the two most common inspection points in the abattoir: 1) with the ante-mortem inspection at the unloading ramp or in the lairage, and 2) with the post-mortem-inspection at the slaughter line. The following list for pigs gives an example of reasonable criteria at the abattoir level that are meaningful for assessing animal health and welfare at herd or flock level:

Recorded by the official veterinarian in the ante-mortem inspection:

- number of lame animals (broken bones, arthritis)
- number of unthrifty and cachectic animals
- number of animals with injuries (acute = transport, and chronic = negligence at farm level)
- number of animals that are not fit for being slaughtered (only due to disease is meaningful)

Recorded by the official veterinarian in the post-mortem inspection:

- number of animals with lesions due to cannibalism (tails, ears)
- number of animals with lesions due to animal cruelty (welts, bruises)
- number of animals that are not fit for consumption due to disease

It is obvious that the criteria listed would change for poultry (food lesions, feather pecking signs, polyserosits etc.), turkey (food lesions, breast blisters, bone deformities etc.) and cattle (mastitis, neglected claws, poor body condition etc.).

Figure 2 demonstrates the principle of benchmarking pig herds using the criteria listed above plus mortality rate and the Antibiotic Treatment Index (the ATI = number of treated animals multiplied by the days of treatment divided by all animals in the herd or flock). Assigning points to each criterion according to the severity of each of the health or welfare impairment will provide the opportunity to calculate for each herd or flock an index that semi-quantitatively measures the quality of the animal health and welfare status. As an example, the mortality rate of finishing pigs could

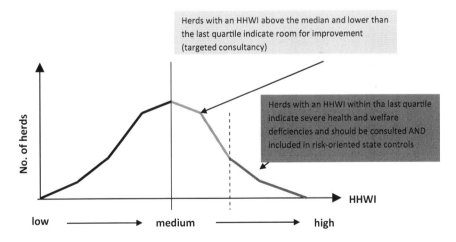

Figure 2. Benchmarking pig herds by measuring their animal health and welfare status by calculating their Herd-Health-Welfare-Index (HHWI) using the same criteria and point system in each of the benchmarked herds.

be graded with points such as: 0 to 1.4% = 0 points, 1.5 to 3.9% = 1 point, 4.0 to 5.9% = 2 points, and >6% = 3 points. All other chosen criteria must be classified in this manner, the points added and the result is the Herd-Health-Welfare-Index (HHWI) specifically developed for each animal species and each cluster of herds or flocks. This method allows for a non-complicated benchmarking of any cluster of comparable food animal production units per animal species.

Such benchmarking systems, applied to pigs, cows, beef cattle, poultry, turkey, etc. would definitely trigger a process of continuous improvement by always identifying herds or flocks that are high, compared to their peer herds and flocks. Figure 3 shows the transition of the way we care for our food animals from curing disease over preventing disease to a systematic animal health and welfare management, which can be accelerated by applying the principles of continuous improvement.

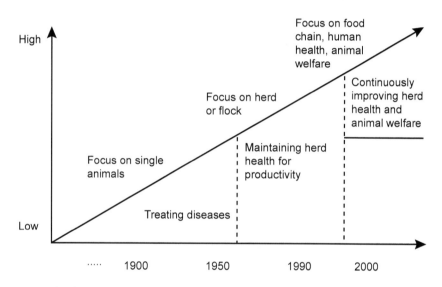

Figure 3. The changes over time in the way animal health, food safety, and animal welfare are guaranteed.

This process will not lead to a complete stop of the current societal criticism with food animal production, but it will considerably contribute to a demonstrable improvement in the conditions under which we keep our food animals and, most of all, how we effectively prevent any suffering of animals and improve their well-being. Another potentially positive side effect of measuring and benchmarking animal health and welfare with animal-oriented indicators of food animal populations will be the generation of health and welfare related data, which can be used to try to "demystify" the myths about the "unavoidable evil" of bigger animal production units and the glorification of small-scale animal holdings.

10

Porcine Reproductive and Respiratory Syndrome Virus and Pig Feed Efficiency and Tissue Accretion

NICHOLAS K. GABLER AND WES SCHWEER

Department of Animal Science, Iowa State University, Ames, IA, USA

Introduction

In pork production, the largest use of natural resources is through the production and consumption of feed. Health-challenged pigs can be a burden on production and pork quality. Therefore, improving feed efficiency and health of pigs is an important goal for sustainable and profitable pork production. The pig is under constant pathogenic challenge which can have adverse effects on intestinal and respiratory health and function, as well as on anabolic processes in peripheral tissues such as skeletal muscle (Williams *et al.*, 1997a, b; Escobar *et al.*, 2004). Of the health challenges the pig industry faces, Porcine Reproductive and Respiratory Syndrome (PRRS) and now Porcine Epidemic Diarrhea (PED) viruses are arguably the two most economically costly viruses to U.S. and world pork production. Alone, PRRS virus infections are estimated to cost the U.S. pig industry more than USD $664 million annually (Holtkamp *et al.*, 2013). In addition to mortality losses and costs of interventions, these viruses may reduce lean tissue accretion and feed efficiency in growing pigs from weaning to market. These reductions may be caused by the innate and adaptive responses to intense, prolonged or poorly contained immunological or stress stimuli. However, single infection alone often fails to induce overt disease; yet they are still recognized individually as important etiological agents in multi-factorial disease of pigs and can negatively impact pig performance. Although it is clearly known that PRRS virus impacts sow reproduction and attenuates average daily gain (ADG) of production pigs, its direct impact on feed efficiency, nutrient and energy digestibility, metabolism and whole body lean and fat accretion in grower / finisher pigs has been poorly characterized.

Immune response to PRRS virus

The PRRS virus is a small, enveloped virus with a single positive-stranded RNA genome, and is a member of the *Arterivirdae* family in the order *Nidovirales* (Albina,

1997). Upon infection and entry into the pig, the virus preferentially replicates in alveolar macrophages, produces a viremia for at least 3-4 weeks, and can persistently infect the lungs, lymphoid tissue and tonsils for up to five months (Albina *et al.*, 1998; Lamontagne *et al.*, 2003). Classically, pigs infected with PRRS virus exhibit a peak serum viremia within 4 to 8 day post inoculation (dpi) and all have serum convert by 14 to 28 dpi (Greiner *et al.*, 2000; Van Gucht *et al.*, 2004; Boddicker *et al.*, 2012; Gabler *et al.*, 2013) (Figure 1). Pigs exposed to PRRS virus have prolonged viremia, often accompanied by persistent infection and virus shedding, and are prone to re-infection and secondary infections.

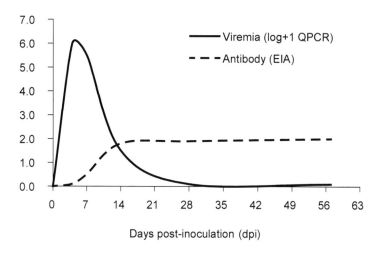

Days post-inoculation (dpi)

Figure 1. Typical PRRS viremia and antibody response in growing pigs (adopted from Greiner *et al.*, 2000; Van Gucht *et al.*, 2004; Boddicker *et al.*, 2012; and Gabler *et al.*, 2013)

A small subset of toll-like receptors (TLR) in the innate immune response are involved in the antiviral response (e.g. TLR 3, 7/8, and 9) and have been shown to produce antiviral cytokines such as type I interferon (IFN). With that, immune dendritic cells (DC) have a unique expression of TLR 7 and 9 which interact with ssRNA or ssDNA and allow rapid type I IFN release after infection (Calzada-Nova *et al.*, 2010). Unlike other arteri-viruses, PRRS virus infection suppresses IFN-α expression by TLR3 thus down regulating IFN-α expression which allows the virus to replicate rapidly (Miller *et al.*, 2009). With that, DCs do not produce IFN-α or TNF-α under PRRS virus infection and these cytokines are important for DC maturation (Calzada-Nova *et al.*, 2010). The blunted and antagonised immune response elicited by PRRS virus may be due to a lack of activation of the transcription factor NF-κB, which is normally activated by TLR regulation through several adaptor molecules or by selectively antagonising activated functions of immune cells (Murtaugh *et al.*, 2002). Although viruses such as PRRS are poor inducers of proinflammatory cytokines, clear evidence from *in vivo* and *in vitro* porcine infection models have shown that pigs infected with PPRS virus are more sensitized to secondary bacterial and viral challenges, and increased proinflammatory cytokine production (Labarque *et al.*, 2002; Van Gucht *et al.*, 2004; Van Gucht *et al.*, 2005). Thus, secondary viral or bacterial challenges leading to dual infection seem to have the greatest effect in early to late nursery phases of growth, and in three site production systems (Dorr *et al.*, 2007). It is often this round of infection that is characterized by a negative nitrogen balance and a decrease in muscle protein content due to increased protein catabolism.

Impact of PRRS on performance and tissue accretion

Although we know that pigs reared in high inflammatory, poor health and dirty conditions can exhibit decreases in protein deposition and growth performance (Williams *et al.*, 1997b), surprisingly there are still little data available that quantifies the true impact PRRS virus has on feed efficiency and tissue accretion in weaner-finisher pigs. Interestingly, Escobar *et al.* (2004) has been the only study to examine the impact of PRRS virus infection on tissue accretion rates. In agreement with Escobar *et al.*, (2004), a significant reduction in ADG, ADFI and feed efficiency in PRRS virus infected pigs has also been reported (Gabler *et al.*, 2013). These reductions are particularly evident within the first four weeks of infection (Figure 2). However, these negative insults on grower-finisher pig production parameters can have a significant effect on lifetime performance (Gabler *et al.*, 2013) (Table 1). This work disagrees with a recent study by Dritz (2012) which reported no difference in weaner or finisher pig feed efficiency in larger commercial U.S. pig operations in the Midwest.

The classical papers (Williams *et al.*, 1997a, b, c) examining poor health immune stimulated pig performance and Escobar *et al.*, (2004) weaned pig-PRRS virus work have been the only major research showing protein accretion is profoundly impacted by immune stimulation. This is particularly evident in the first week of PRRS virus infection where whole protein accretion is impeded by up to 60% from naïve control pigs and by 33% in week 2 (Escobar *et al.*, 2004). A longitudinal assessment of body composition using dual X-ray absorptiometry on the same pig (not using the traditional serial slaughter technique), indicated that protein accretion was impeded by 24% in the first 42 dpi and by 5% in the following 35 days; overall, this resulted in a 10% reduction in protein accretion over an 80 dpi period (Table 1; Gabler *et al.*, 2013). Similarly, non-pathogenic lipopolysaccharide (LPS) challenge models have also been shown to decrease acutely muscle protein synthesis *in vivo* and *in vitro* through impaired phosphorylation of both eIF4E-binding protein 1 (4E-BP1) and ribosomal protein S6 kinase 1 (S6K1) in the mammalian target of rapamycin (mTOR) pathway, which is a key determinant of translation initiation

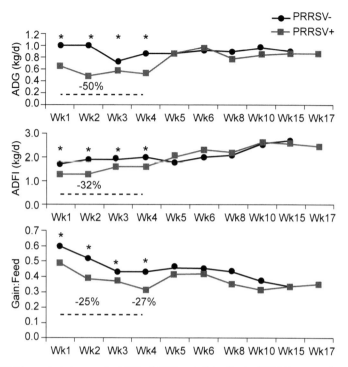

Figure 2. Within period changes in ADG, ADFI and Gain:Feed of PRRS virus infected and naïve gilts. n=5 pen/trt, * P < 0.05 within period.

Table 1. Performance of gilts infected with PRRS virus or without (CONT) from _35-127 kg BW_.

Parameter	CONT	PRRSv	SE	P-value
[1]Performance, 0-112 dpi				
ADG, kg/d	0.89	0.80	0.032	<0.05
ADFI, kg/d	2.05	1.93	0.058	<0.05
Feed:Gain	2.30	2.41	0.026	<0.05
[2]Tissue Accretion, 0-80				
Lean, g/d	657	568	13.9	<0.001
Protein, g/d	131	112	2.89	<0.001
Fat, g/d	230	184	9.22	<0.001
Bone, g/d	27.8	26.0	0.94	0.063
[3]Apparent total tract digestibility (coefficient), 19-21 dpi				
Dry matter	0.839	0.813	0.0054	<0.001
Nitrogen	0.818	0.773	0.0084	<0.001
Energy	0.810	0.778	0.0064	<0.001
[2]Carcass yield, %	76.7	75.4		
[2]Carcass lean, %	55.4	56.3		
[2]Carcass backfat depth, cm	1.85	1.50		
[2]Carcass loin depth, cm	7.00	7.00		

[1]n=6 gilts per treatment
[2]n=30 gilts per treatment
[3]n=15 gilts per treatment

and protein synthesis in pigs (Kimball *et al.*, 2002, 2003; Orellana *et al.*, 2007a, b). This inhibition of the translation initiation process seems to be a direct effect of the inflammatory response, but the subsequent increase in proinflammatory cytokines may augment the depression in protein synthesis events and rates (Lang *et al.*, 2002, 2003, 2007; Lang and Frost, 2007). Also observed has been a reduced whole body lipid accretion rates (Table 1) due to PRRS virus infection by up to 20% compared to healthy PRRS naïve littermates (Gabler *et al.*, 2013). Altogether, these data translated into leaner pigs at market weight and reduced yields (Table 1). Reduced carcass yields are probably the result of higher offal and internal organ weights associated with immune stimulated pigs (Williams *et al.*, 1997c; Rakhshandeh and de Lange, 2012).

Based on a recent meta-analysis of pig microarray studies, innate and adaptive responses to intense, prolonged and poorly-contained immunological stimuli are most probably responsible for reductions in performance (Badaoui *et al.*, 2013). This meta-analysis revealed mitochondrial dysfunction and oxidative phosphorylation pathways to be activated by PRRS virus infection. Infections by pathogens have been shown to alter cell homeostasis and cause an elevation in cellular reactive oxygen species (ROS) via mitochondrial dysfunction (Chakraborty *et al.*, 2012a, b). However, the role of PRRS virus infection in augmenting mitochondrial dysfunction and ROS production is not known, but may be related to decreases in feed efficiencies in health challenged animals. Further studies (Grubbs *et al.*, 2013a, b) and others (Bottje *et al.*, 2002; Iqbal *et al.*, 2004; Ojano-Dirain *et al.*, 2007) have previously reported that mitochondrial inefficiency may occur as a result of electron leakage and contribute to the phenotypic expression of low feed efficiency. Therefore, poor nutrient and energy utilization by livestock under disease challenge may be accounted for by changes in mechanisms responsible for regulation of mitochondria function. Elevated mitochondrial ROS from electron leakage can cause the diversion of dietary energy from growth and development processes towards cellular repair and/or autophagy mechanisms.

Another key component that has been poorly defined in meat animal production is the direct link between mitochondrial function, proteolysis and protein turnover. It is estimated that protein turnover and tissue metabolism accounts for 37% of the variation in residual feed intake in beef cattle (Richardson and Herd, 2004). Protein turnover based on the independent roles and regulation of protein degradation and synthesis, is known to be energetically expensive and may account for ~20% of the increase in ATP expenditure in sheep (Gill *et al.*, 1989). ROS production increases protein carbonyl formation, which has been reported by Bottje (2006) to increase in low feed efficiency (FE; gain:feed) broiler tissues. Importantly, these proteins may be more susceptible to degradation. Due to the proximity of the electron transport chain (ETC) to sites of mitochondrial ROS production, and that many ETC proteins have reactive protein thiols, ETC proteins are particularly vulnerable to oxidation. Ojano-

Dirain et al., (2005) did report positive correlations between reduced glutathione (GSH, an important mitochondrial antioxidant) and activities of Complex II, IV and V, indicating antioxidant protection is important in optimal activity of the ETC. Acute mitochondrial insults from stress, viruses and inflammation can impair mitochondrial function leading to cellular energetic depression, ROS production and intracellular Ca^{2+} overload (Seppet et al., 2009). Moreover, the link between mitochondrial function, oxidative stress and protein degradation is closely linked with intracellular Ca^{2+} homeostasis and the activity of calpain, a family of calcium (Ca^{2+})-dependent cysteine proteases (Lu et al., 2013). Sepsis, viremia and inflammation are all associated with a pronounced catabolic response in skeletal muscle. Conversely, sepsis has been shown to release myofilaments from myofibrillar proteins in a calcium-dependent manner (Williams et al., 1999).

Protein degradation pathways such as the µ- and m-calpain and calpastatin system and the ubiquitin-proteasome pathway, may play a role in FE and are known to contribute to protein turnover through protein degradation in muscle (Smith and Dodd, 2007). In the ubiquitin-proteasome pathway, proteins selected for degradation are poly-ubiquitinated tagged in an ATP dependent manner and then presented to the proteasome where proteolysis occurs. Differences in protein ubiquination in broilers divergent in FE have been reported (Bottje and Carstens, 2009). We have recently reported substantial evidence that these protein degradation systems (µ- and m-calpain, and 20S proteasome activities) within muscle are increased in less FE pigs (Cruzen et al., 2013). The proteasome is a multi-catalytic complex in the nucleus and cytosol of all eukaryotic cells that is responsible for proteolysis of ubiquitin-tagged proteins. This system primarily breaks down structural proteins which are further degraded to small peptide fragments and free amino acids by the ubiquitin-proteasome system. The 20S subunit is the catalytic core of the 26S proteasome with two 19S regulatory caps. The 20S core is where proteins are degraded and the 19S regulatory caps have multiple ATPase active sites and ubiquitin binding sites to recognize polyubiquinated proteins to be transferred to the catalytic core (Voges et al., 1999).

Alternatively, calpastatin inhibits the calpain system from degrading proteins of larger myofibrillar proteins. Desmin, an intermediate filament that links adjacent myofibrils, can also undergo rapid proteolysis. Since postmortem protein degradation is what creates tender meat, an increase in calpastatin activity and intact desmin would indicate a decrease in meat tenderness. We have also reported that pigs selected for improved feed efficiency have higher calpastatin activity in the loin muscle and intact desmin has been shown to have a negative correlation with RFI (Smith et al., 2011). Interestingly, Escobar et al., (2004) have shown that nursery pigs infected with PRRS virus had reduced protein accretion over a 28 day period and increases in mRNA abundance of myostatin. Myostatin is a negative regulator of muscle mass in mammalian species and is capable of inducing muscle atrophy under stress, sepsis and inflammatory conditions via the inhibition of myoblast proliferation and increasing ubiquitin-proteasomal activity (Elliott *et al.*, 2012). Additionally, preliminary data from Dr. Steven Lonergan in conjunction with our laboratory is showing PRRS virus infection to increase skeletal muscle calpain activity and inhibit calpastatin activities compared to PRRS naïve muscle samples. Collectively, it is assumed that the associated growth depression and diversion of nutrients away from tissue accretion ensures adequate energy and nutrients are available for high priority immunological and homeostatic pathways. However, overall protein degradation and turnover has also been poorly characterized in poor health livestock.

Impact of health challenges on digestibility

Poor health pigs also often exhibit reduced appetite and feed intake and altered nutrient utilization in a tissue-specific manner (Johnson, 2002). However, this impact on nutrient digestibility in the face of PRRS virus is poorly characterized. Interestingly, the impact of immune stimulation of nutrient and energy digestibility has also been poorly described, particularly using industry applicable pathogens. Lipopolysaccharide (LPS) has been extensively used to study the inflammatory response in pigs. More recently, repeated challenges with LPS have been used to mimic pathogenic challenges like PRRS virus (Rakhshandeh and de Lange, 2012; Rakhshandeh *et al.*, 2012a); these studies have shown that inflammation reduces apparent total tract digestibility (ATTD) of organic matter, energy and nitrogen. Similarly, at 21 dpi it was clearly shown that ATTD of nitrogen, dry matter and energy was reduced due to PRRS virus infection (Table 1). Significantly, this attenuation of total tract digestibility may be long-lasting and can still be seen at 70 dpi (Unpublished data). However, at this stage it can only be speculated these are a result of intestinal microbial population alterations or changes endogenous secretions of proteins such as mucins.

The observed decrease in ATTD of nitrogen seen in LPS and PRRS challenge models could potentially be described by an increase in endogenous secretions of mucus into the lumen. Although tight junction proteins are important barrier defences, changes in intestinal transepithelial resistance (integrity marker) in pigs under sustained LPS induced inflammation are not seen (Rakhshandeh *et al.*, 2012b). The mucus layer coating the length of the intestinal tract provides the first line of defence against intestinal injury, and allows for nutrient transport while at the same time preventing microbial attachment and colonization (Kim and Ho, 2010). Intestinal goblet cells are responsible for secretion of several homeostatic mucins (MUC) including MUC1, MUC2, MUC 3, MUC4, MUC 12, MUC 13, and MUC17 (Johansson *et al.*, 2013). MUC5AC secretion has been reported to be augmented in response to inflammatory conditions (Wilberts *et al.*, 2014). Mucins are large glycosylated glycoproteins enriched with threonine with several O-linked oligosaccharide side chains, which create a gel-like structure (Kim and Ho, 2010). Several factors including microbes, microbial products, cytokines, toxins, and more regulate expression of mucin genes. The mucus layer also contains several other products including trefoil factors (TFF), antimicrobial peptides (β-defensins, lysozymes) and secretory IgA. Resistin-like molecule β is also secreted by goblet cells and induces goblet cell hyperplasia as well as functions as an immune effector molecule in response to a nematode infection (Johansson *et al.*, 2009). Thus, these secretory compounds may have a profound impact on intestinal integrity and amino acid metabolism during a disease or inflammatory challenge.

Health challenges and metabolism

Both the innate and adaptive immune responses are integrated with cellular bioenergetics, metabolism, and inflammation at a whole animal, tissue and cellular levels. However, there is still minimal knowledge on how PRRS virus infection may regulation a pig's metabolism. By understanding the metabolic ramifications of these viral infections, better mitigation strategies can be employed to reduce the severity of health challenges to pig and business performance. Homeorhetic switches in bioenergy intimately links metabolism with immune function and inflammation to restore homeostasis and protect cells. Profound metabolic reprogramming occurs in which there is a heightened reliance on glycolysis and a down regulation of oxidative phosphorylation (O'Neill, 2011; Tannahill *et al.*, 2013). Specifically, Tannahill *et al.*, (2013) reported that the activation of Toll-like receptors in the innate immune response leads to a switch from oxidative phosphorylation to glycolytic; it was stated that glycolysis and glucose metabolism is preferred so the cell can generate more ATP per unit time for immune and homeostatic needs, even though it is not as efficient in terms of ATP generation as the process of oxidative phosphorylation in mitochondria.

The way cells and tissue perceive and respond to an immune challenge can result in metabolic polarities (Liu *et al.*, 2012). The initiating proinflammatory phase in response to infection and inflammation is anabolic and requires glucose as the primary fuel, whereas the opposing adaptation phase is catabolic and requires fatty acid oxidation (McCall *et al.*, 2011). Early glycolytic reprogramming provides a surge of ATP under normoxia conditions, thereby simulating the Warburg effect of glycolysis and reduced mitochondrial glucose oxidation as typically seen in many cancer cells (Lu *et al.*, 2014). Glycolysis also activates the pentose shunt to kill bacteria by NADPH oxidase and increased ROS production. The regulatory components of augmented glucose fueling include increased expression glucose transporters and glycolysis regulatory genes, and disrupted mitochondrial glucose oxidation by pyruvate dehydrogenase kinase (PDHK), which deactivates mitochondrial pyruvate dehydrogenase. This in turn limits mitochondrial glucose oxidation, increasing intracellular and extracellular pyruvate and lactate. The glycolysis surge and reduced glucose mitochondrial oxidation is hypoxia (HIF-1α) dependent, which is transactivated via stabilized by inactivating prolyl hydroxylase activity by inflammatory NF-κB and other signaling events (O'Neill and Hardie, 2013; Lu *et al.*, 2014). Critically, increased glucose flux is required for immunocompetent effector responses. The increase in aerobic glycolysis allows the TCA cycle to provide precursors for biosynthesis, rather than ATP production. Additionally, the buildup TCA cycle intermediates such as citrate and succinate may act as inflammatory signals (O'Neill, 2011; Tannahill *et al.*, 2013).

Infection also causes a state of pseudo-starvation due to suppressed feed intake and increase energetic demands. This is evented during the adaptation phase to infection and inflammation which is more catabolic and requires fatty acid oxidation (Liu *et al.*, 2012). Activation of AMP-activated protein kinase (AMPK) would promote the switch to an anti-inflammatory phenotype and cause a switch away from glycolysis towards mitochondrial oxidative phosphorylation and fatty acid oxidation (O'Neill and Hardie, 2013). Interestingly, AMPK-mediated pathways have been shown to be involved in the antiviral response to PRRS virus infection (Sang *et al.*, 2014). Immuno-metabolism, metabolic homeostasis and homeorhesis is a relatively new frontier that focuses on the integration and interaction of immune and metabolic systems. This work in meat livestock species is limited. However, by understanding the metabolic pathways activated and the coordinated hormonal response (insulin, glucagon, etc) to infection, metabolism targeted interventions and management strategies for poor health livestock could be developed to mitigate production losses. These advances will enhance lean tissue and feed efficiency of pigs that can also be extended to other species to enhance global food security and sustainability.

Conclusion

In summary, this ongoing project is clearly demonstrating that PRRS virus infection reduces not only ADG, but also ADFI, coefficients of apparent total tract digestibility, and feed efficiency in grow-finisher gilts. Furthermore, lean/protein and fat accretion rates all appear to be affected to a similar extent. Additional blood analysis and carcass data from this project will allow us to better understand the metabolic impact of PRRS virus in pigs and to calculate the economic impact of this health challenge in a grow-finisher production setting. Based on this data set, overall we conservatively estimated the economic impact of PRRS virus to cost the producer between USD$6.14 - USD$12.85 per head.

Acknowledgements

This paper has been supported by funds from the National Pork Board grant #12-163; Choice Genetics, West Des Moines, IA, USA; the Agriculture and Food Research Initiative Competitive Grant no. 2011-68004-30336 from the USDA National Institute of Food and Agriculture; and funds form the Animal Health and Disease Research Capacity Grant Program, by State of Iowa funds.

References

Albina, E. (1997) Epidemiology of porcine reproductive and respiratory syndrome (PRRS): An overview. *Veterinary Microbiology,* **55**, 309-316.

Albina, E., L. Piriou, E. Hutet, R. Cariolet, and R. L'Hospitalier. (1998) Immune responses in pigs infected with porcine reproductive and respiratory syndrome virus (PRRSV). *Veterinary Immunology and Immunopathology,* **61**, 49-66.

Badaoui, B., C. K. Tuggle, Z. Hu, J. M. Reecy, T. Ait-Ali, A. Anselmo, and S. Botti. (2013) Pig immune response to general stimulus and to porcine reproductive and respiratory syndrome virus infection: a meta-analysis approach. *BMC genomics,* **14**, 220.

Boddicker, N., E. H. Waide, R. R. Rowland, J. K. Lunney, D. J. Garrick, J. M. Reecy, and J. C. Dekkers. (2012) Evidence for a major QTL associated with host response to porcine reproductive and respiratory syndrome virus challenge. *J Anim Sci,* **90**, 1733-1746.

Bottje, W., M. Iqbal, Z. X. Tang, D. Cawthon, R. Okimoto, T. Wing, and M. Cooper. (2002) Association of mitochondrial function with feed efficiency within a single genetic line of male broilers. *Poultry Science,* **81**, 546-555.

Bottje, W., N. R. Pumford, C. Ojano-Dirain, M. Iqbal, and K. Lassiter. (2006) Feed efficiency and mitochondrial function. *Poultry Science,* **85**, 8-14.

Bottje, W. G., and G. E. Carstens. (2009) Association of mitochondrial function and feed efficiency in poultry and livestock species. *J Anim Sci,* **87**, E48-63.

Calzada-Nova, G., W. Schnitzlein, R. Husmann, and F. A. Zuckermann. (2010) Characterization of the cytokine and maturation responses of pure populations of porcine plasmacytoid dendritic cells to porcine viruses and toll-like receptor agonists. *Vet Immunol Immunopathol,* **135**, 20-33.

Chakraborty, S. P., S. Das, S. Chattopadhyay, S. Tripathy, S. K. Dash, P. Pramanik, and S. Roy. (2012a) Staphylococcus aureus infection induced redox signaling and DNA fragmentation in T-lymphocytes: possible ameliorative role of nanoconjugated vancomycin. *Toxicology Mechanisms and Methods,* **22**, 193-204.

Chakraborty, S. P., P. Pramanik, and S. Roy. (2012b) Staphylococcus aureus Infection Induced Oxidative Imbalance in Neutrophils: Possible Protective Role of Nanoconjugated Vancomycin. *ISRN Pharmacology,* **2012**, 435214.

Cruzen, S. M., A. J. Harris, K. Hollinger, R. M. Punt, J. K. Grubbs, J. T. Selsby, J. C. Dekkers, N. K. Gabler, S. M. Lonergan, and E. Huff-Lonergan. (2013) Evidence of decreased muscle protein turnover in gilts selected for low residual feed intake. *J Anim Sci,* **91**, 4007-4016.

Dorr, P. M., R. B. Baker, G. W. Almond, S. R. Wayne, and W. A. Gebreyes. (2007) Epidemiologic assessment of porcine circovirus type 2 coinfection with other pathogens in swine. *J Am Vet Med Assoc,* **230**, 244-250.

Dritz, S. S. (2012) Influence of health on feed efficiency. In: J. F. Patience (ed.) *Feed efficiency in swine.* p 225-237. Wageningen Academic Publishers.

Elliott, B., D. Renshaw, S. Getting, and R. Mackenzie. (2012) The central role of myostatin in skeletal muscle and whole body homeostasis. *Acta Physiol (Oxf),* **205**, 324-340.

Escobar, J., W. G. Van Alstine, D. H. Baker, and R. W. Johnson. (2004) Decreased protein accretion in pigs with viral and bacterial pneumonia is associated with increased myostatin expression in muscle. *J Nutr,* **134**, 3047-3053.

Gabler, N. K., W. Schweer, J. F. Patience, L. Karriker, J. C. Sparks, G. Gourley, M. FitzSimmons, K. Schwartz, and T. E. Burkey. (2013) The impact of PRRSV on feed efficiency, digestibility and tissue accretion in grow-finisher pigs. Allen D. Leman Swine Conference. No. 40. p 135-136. Veterinary Continuing Education, St. Paul, Mn, USA.

Gill, M., J. France, M. Summers, B. W. McBride, and L. P. Milligan. (1989) Simulation of the energy costs associated with protein-turnover and Na+,K+-transport in growing lambs. *J Nutr,* **119**, 1287-1299.

Greiner, L. L., T. S. Stahly, and T. J. Stabel. (2000) Quantitative relationship of systemic virus concentration on growth and immune response in pigs. *J Anim Sci,* **78**, 2690-2695.

Grubbs, J. K., A. N. Fritchen, E. Huff-Lonergan, J. C. Dekkers, N. K. Gabler, and S. M. Lonergan. (2013a) Divergent genetic selection for residual feed intake impacts mitochondria reactive oxygen species production in pigs. *J Anim Sci,* **91**, 2133-2140.

Grubbs, J. K., A. N. Fritchen, E. Huff-Lonergan, N. K. Gabler, and S. M. Lonergan. (2013b) Selection for residual feed intake alters the mitochondria protein profile in pigs. *Journal of Proteomics,* **80**, 334-345.

Holtkamp, D. J., J. B. Kliebenstein, E. J. Neumann, J. J. Zimmerman, H. F. Rotto, T. K. Yoder, C. Wang, P. E. Yeske, C. L. Mowrer, and C. A. Haley. (2013) Assessment of the economic impact of porcine reproductive and respiratory syndrome virus on United States pork producers. *Journal of Swine Health and Production,* **21**, 72-84.

Iqbal, M., N. R. Pumford, Z. X. Tang, K. Lassiter, T. Wing, M. Cooper, and W. Bottje. (2004) Low feed efficient broilers within a single genetic line exhibit higher oxidative stress and protein expression in breast muscle with lower mitochondrial complex activity. *Poultry Science,* **83**, 474-484.

Johansson, M. E., H. Sjovall, and G. C. Hansson. (2013) The gastrointestinal mucus system in health and disease. Nature reviews. *Gastroenterology & Hepatology,* **10**, 352-361.

Johansson, M. E., K. A. Thomsson, and G. C. Hansson. (2009) Proteomic analyses of the two mucus layers of the colon barrier reveal that their main component, the Muc2 mucin, is strongly bound to the Fcgbp protein. *Journal of Proteome Research,* **8**, 3549-3557.

Johnson, R. W. (2002) The concept of sickness behavior: a brief chronological account of four key discoveries. *Veterinary Immunology and Immunopathology,* **87**, 443-450.

Kim, Y. S., and S. B. Ho. (2010) Intestinal goblet cells and mucins in health and disease: recent insights and progress. *Current Gastroenterology Reports,* **12**, 319-330.

Kimball, S. R., P. A. Farrell, H. V. Nguyen, L. S. Jefferson, and T. A. Davis. (2002) Developmental decline in components of signal transduction pathways regulating protein synthesis in pig muscle. *Am J Physiol Endocrinol Metab,* **282**, E585-592.

Kimball, S. R., R. A. Orellana, P. M. O'Connor, A. Suryawan, J. A. Bush, H. V. Nguyen, M. C. Thivierge, L. S. Jefferson, and T. A. Davis. (2003) Endotoxin induces differential regulation of mTOR-dependent signaling in skeletal muscle and liver of neonatal pigs. *Am J Physiol Endocrinol Metab,* **285**, E637-644.

Labarque, G., K. Van Reeth, S. Van Gucht, H. Nauwynck, and M. Pensaert. (2002) Porcine reproductive-respiratory syndrome virus infection predisposes pigs for respiratory signs upon exposure to bacterial lipopolysaccharide. *Vet Microbiol,* **88**, 1-12.

Lamontagne, L., C. Page, R. Larochelle, and R. Magar. (2003) Porcine reproductive and respiratory syndrome virus persistence in blood, spleen, lymph nodes, and tonsils of experimentally infected pigs depends on the level of CD8(high) T cells. *Viral Immunology,* **16**, 395-406.

Lang, C. H., and R. A. Frost. (2007) Sepsis-induced suppression of skeletal muscle translation initiation mediated by tumor necrosis factor alpha. *Metabolism,* **56**, 49-57.

Lang, C. H., R. A. Frost, A. C. Nairn, D. A. MacLean, and T. C. Vary. (2002) TNF-alpha impairs heart and skeletal muscle protein synthesis by altering translation initiation. *Am. J. Physiol. Endocrinol. Metab,* **282**, E336-347.

Lang, C. H., R. A. Frost, and T. C. Vary. (2007) Regulation of Muscle Protein Synthesis During Sepsis and Inflammation. *Am J Physiol Endocrinol Metab.*

Lang, C. H., C. Silvis, N. Deshpande, G. Nystrom, and R. A. Frost. (2003) Endotoxin stimulates in vivo expression of inflammatory cytokines tumor necrosis factor alpha, interleukin-1beta, -6, and high-mobility-group protein-1 in skeletal muscle. *Shock,* **19**, 538-546.

Liu, T. F., C. M. Brown, M. El Gazzar, L. McPhail, P. Millet, A. Rao, V. T. Vachharajani, B. K. Yoza, and C. E. McCall. (2012) Fueling the flame: bioenergy couples metabolism and inflammation. *Journal of Leukocyte Biology,* **92**, 499-507.

Lu, J., M. Tan, and Q. Cai. (2014) The Warburg effect in tumor progression: Mitochondrial oxidative metabolism as an anti-metastasis mechanism. *Cancer letters.*

Lu, J. R., W. W. Lu, J. Z. Lai, F. L. Tsai, S. H. Wu, C. W. Lin, and S. H. Kung. (2013) Calcium flux and calpain-mediated activation of the apoptosis-inducing factor contribute to enterovirus 71-induced apoptosis. *The Journal of General Virology,* **94**, 1477-1485.

McCall, C. E., M. El Gazzar, T. Liu, V. Vachharajani, and B. Yoza. (2011) Epigenetics, bioenergetics, and microRNA coordinate gene-specific reprogramming during acute systemic inflammation. *Journal of Leukocyte Biology,* **90**, 439-446.

Miller, L. C., K. M. Lager, and M. E. Kehrli, Jr. (2009) Role of Toll-like receptors in activation of porcine alveolar macrophages by porcine reproductive and respiratory syndrome virus. *Clinical and vaccine immunology : CVI,* **16**, 360-365.

Murtaugh, M. P., Z. Xiao, and F. Zuckermann. (2002) Immunological responses of swine to porcine reproductive and respiratory syndrome virus infection. *Viral Immunol,* **15**, 533-547.

O'Neill, L. A. (2011) A critical role for citrate metabolism in LPS signalling. *The Biochemical Journal,* **438**, e5-6.

O'Neill, L. A., and D. G. Hardie. (2013) Metabolism of inflammation limited by AMPK and pseudo-starvation. *Nature,* **493**, 346-355.

Ojano-Dirain, C., M. Iqbal, T. Wing, M. Cooper, and W. Bottje. (2005) Glutathione and respiratory chain complex activity in duodenal mitochondria of broilers with low and high feed efficiency. *Poultry Science,* **84**, 782-788.

Ojano-Dirain, C., N. B. Tinsley, T. Wing, M. Cooper, and W. G. Bottje. (2007) Membrane potential and H_2O_2 production in duodenal mitochondria from broiler chickens (Gallus gallus domesticus) with low and high feed efficiency. *Comparative biochemistry and physiology. Part A, Molecular & integrative physiology,* **147**, 934-941.

Orellana, R. A., A. Jeyapalan, J. Escobar, J. W. Frank, H. V. Nguyen, A. Suryawan, and T. A. Davis. (2007a) Amino acids augment muscle protein synthesis in neonatal pigs during acute endotoxemia by stimulating mTOR-dependent translation initiation. *Am J Physiol Endocrinol Metab,* **293**, E1416-1425.

Orellana, R. A., S. R. Kimball, A. Suryawan, J. Escobar, H. V. Nguyen, L. S. Jefferson, and T. A. Davis. 2007b. Insulin stimulates muscle protein synthesis in neonates during endotoxemia despite repression of translation initiation. *Am J Physiol Endocrinol Metab,* **292**, E629-636.

Rakhshandeh, A., and C. F. de Lange. (2012) Evaluation of chronic immune system stimulation models in growing pigs. *Animal : an International Journal of Animal Bioscience,* **6**, 305-310.

Rakhshandeh, A., J. Dekkers, B. Kerr, T. Weber, J. English, and N. Gabler. (2012a) Effect of immune system stimulation and divergent selection for residual feed intake on digestive capacity of the small intestine in growing pigs. *Journal of Animal Science,* **90**, 233-235.

Rakhshandeh, A., J. C. M. Dekkers, B. J. Kerr, T. E. Weber, J. English, and N. K. Gabler. (2012b) Effect of immune system stimulation and divergent selection for residual feed intake on digestive capacity of the small intestine in growing pigs. *J Anim Sci,* **90**, 233-235.

Richardson, E. C., and R. M. Herd. (2004) Biological basis for variation in residual feed intake in beef cattle. 2. Synthesis of results following divergent selection. *Aust J Exp Agr,* **44**, 431-440.

Sang, Y., W. Brichalli, R. R. Rowland, and F. Blecha. (2014) Genome-wide analysis of antiviral signature genes in porcine macrophages at different activation statuses. *PloS one,* **9**, e87613.

Seppet, E. *et al.* (2009) Mitochondria and energetic depression in cell pathophysiology. *International Journal of Molecular Sciences,* **10**, 2252-2303.

Smith, I. J., and S. L. Dodd. (2007) Calpain activation causes a proteasome-dependent increase in protein degradation and inhibits the Akt signalling pathway in rat diaphragm muscle. *Experimental Physiology,* **92**, 561-573.

Smith, R. M., N. K. Gabler, J. M. Young, W. Cai, N. J. Boddicker, M. J. Anderson, E. Huff-Lonergan, J. C. Dekkers, and S. M. Lonergan. (2011) Effects of selection for decreased residual feed intake on composition and quality of fresh pork. *J Anim Sci,* **89**, 192-200.

Tannahill, G. M. *et al.* (2013) Succinate is an inflammatory signal that induces IL-1beta through HIF-1alpha. *Nature,* **496**, 238-242.

Van Gucht, S., G. Labarque, and K. Van Reeth. (2004) The combination of PRRS virus and bacterial endotoxin as a model for multifactorial respiratory disease in pigs. *Vet Immunol Immunopathol,* **102**, 165-178.

Van Gucht, S., K. Van Reeth, H. Nauwynck, and M. Pensaert. (2005) Porcine reproductive and respiratory syndrome virus infection increases CD14 expression and lipopolysaccharide-binding protein in the lungs of pigs. *Viral Immunol,* **18**, 116-126.

Voges, D., P. Zwickl, and W. Baumeister. (1999) The 26S proteasome: A molecular machine designed for controlled proteolysis. *Annu. Rev. Biochem,* **68**, 1015-1068.

Wilberts, B. L., P. H. Arruda, J. M. Kinyon, D. M. Madson, T. S. Frana, and E. R. Burrough. (2014) Comparison of Lesion Severity, Distribution, and Colonic Mucin Expression in Pigs With Acute Swine Dysentery Following Oral Inoculation With "Brachyspira hampsonii" or Brachyspira hyodysenteriae. *Veterinary pathology.*

Williams, A. B., G. M. Decourten-Myers, J. E. Fischer, G. Luo, X. Sun, and P. O. Hasselgren. (1999) Sepsis stimulates release of myofilaments in skeletal muscle by a calcium-dependent mechanism. *The FASEB journal : official publication of the Federation of American Societies for Experimental Biology,* **13**, 1435-1443.

Williams, N. H., T. S. Stahly, and D. R. Zimmerman. (1997a) Effect of chronic immune system activation on body nitrogen retention, partial efficiency of lysine utilization, and lysine needs of pigs. *J Anim Sci,* **75**, 2472-2480.

Williams, N. H., T. S. Stahly, and D. R. Zimmerman. (1997b) Effect of chronic immune system activation on the rate, efficiency, and composition of growth and lysine needs of pigs fed from 6 to 27 kg. *J Anim Sci,* **75**, 2463-2471.

Williams, N. H., T. S. Stahly, and D. R. Zimmerman. (1997c) Effect of level of chronic immune system activation on the growth and dietary lysine needs of pigs fed from 6 to 112 kg. *J Anim Sci,* **75**, 2481-2496.

11

More Pigs Born Per Sow Per Year – Feeding and Management of the Bottom 20% of the Pig Population

PETE WILCOCK[1] AND IAN WELLOCK[2]

[1]*AB Vista, UK;* [2]*Primary Diets*

There is a current focus on increasing pork output per sow per year and this is resulting in a greater emphasis on targeting more pigs per sow per year. This is mainly being driven by an increase in litter size which can have negative effect on birth and weaning weights as well as subsequent pig performance. This paper will look at the implications that litter size has on birth and weaning weights and subsequent pig performance. In addition it will review some of the main nutritional and management practices that can be used to assist weaning and post-weaning performance. It is not within the scope of this paper to do a detailed review of this whole topic but rather focus on some key elements of improving the bottom 20% pig performance.

Increasing litter size

In most key markets there has been a large increase in the number of pigs born alive per litter and in Denmark they are now targeting 35 pigs weaned per sow per year. In the USA there has been a mean litter size increase of 1.2 pigs born alive since 2005 with the top ten percent of the market increasing litter size by almost 1.5 pigs born live (Figure 1). This drive for greater litter size improves financial return as the pork marketed per sow per year increases while the cost per weaned pig is reduced. Indeed a combination of greater pigs weaned per sow and heavier slaughter weights make the 4 tonne per sow target already achievable in some of the top units in the USA. This increased litter size can however come at a cost with smaller birthweights leading to an increased level of mortality (pre-weaning and lifetime) as well as poorer growth performance post-weaning. Management and nutritional practices that can assist the small piglet performance have become more important in maximizing pork output per sow.

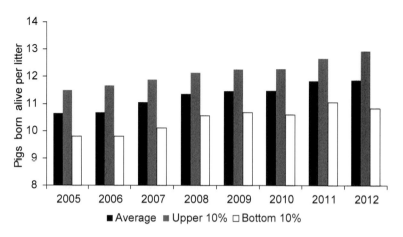

Figure 1. Average Pigs Born Alive Per Litter (USA) (Pig Champ, 2005 - 2012)

Birthweight

With the target of greater litter size being the focus it has resulted in what is believed to be uterine crowding that can result in lower birthweights and subsequent performance. It has been suggested (Foxcroft, 2006 and Berard *et al.*, 2010) that with the hyper-prolific sow there is a greater ovulation rate and by day 30 of gestation there are an increased level of conceptus surviving which has a negative impact on placental development and uterine crowding in this period. This limits nutrient utilisation during a critical developmental period of the embryo. Although at day 50 the number of conceptuses has been reduced, the placental development is still impaired resulting in poor foetus growth and a reduced level of muscle fibres at birth. This is believed to have a negative effect on birthweight and subsequent animal performance as well as negatively impacting pork quality.

Contrary to the earlier findings that lower birthweights can negatively impact carcass characteristics as well as birthweights, research by Beaulieu *et al.* (2010) showed that there was no negative effect of birthweight on carcass analyses or eating quality. However the data did confirm that increasing litter size reduced average birthweight and that birthweight affected the subsequent pig performance with the lightest birthweight pigs taking 10 days longer to get to market (Table 1). The differences in studies regarding the impact of birthweight on carcass analyses and eating quality may be attributed to the genetic line used.

The impact that birthweight can have on subsequent performance and lifetime full value pigs was shown in a commercial research study conducted by Boyd (2012). In this study, data of 6039 piglets was collected at birth and there was an inverse

Table 1. Effect of birthweight on days to market

	Birthweight (kg)					
	0.75 to 1.20	1.25 to 1.45	1.50 to 1.70	1.75 to 2.50	SEM	P-value
Shipping weight	119.31	119.23	119.68	119.47	0.39	0.78
Mean days to market	159.3a	154.9b	152.3c	149.6d	0.80	<0.001

Note: Adapted from Beaulieu *et al.* (2010)

relationship between increasing litter size and mean birthweight (Figure 2). This reduced mean birthweight also resulted in a higher percentage of small piglets. As an example increasing pigs born alive from 10 to 13 pigs resulted in a mean drop in birthweight of 0.12 kg but more importantly increased the percentage of pigs less than 1.13 kg from 12% to 17.6%.

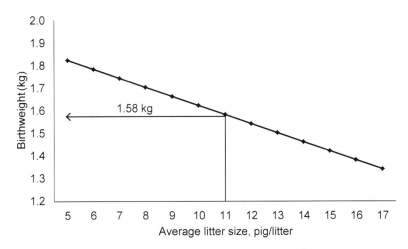

Figure 2. Relationship between litter size born alive and piglet birthweight (Boyd, 2012)

The impact that this can have on subsequent performance is dramatic and Boyd (2012) showed (Figure. 3) in a second study that to optimise pre-weaning mortality (PWM), wean-finish mortality (WFM) and life time full value (FV) in pigs (percent of pigs that were born alive and survived to market) the optimal birthweight was > 1.58 kg. This birthweight from the initial study (Figure 2) would relate to 11 pigs born alive and so any increase in litter size above this would have a detrimental effect on PWM, WFM and FV based on these two studies. This data was confirmed by Fix and See (2009) when in a study of 5252 piglets they showed that there was no improvement in pre-weaning mortality in piglets that were greater than 1.5 kg in birthweight and that reducing birthweight has a negative effect on growth. In general, targeting a birthweight of 1.5 kg or greater would be beneficial although this may differ somewhat between genetic lines.

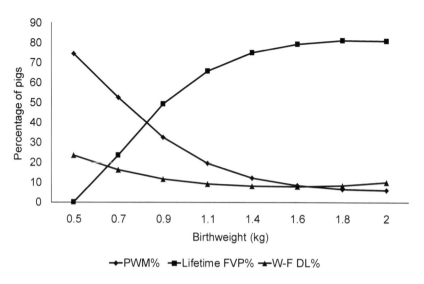

Figure 3. Effect of birthweight on pre-weaning mortality (PWM), wean-finish mortality (W-F-DL%) and life-time full value pigs (FVP) at slaughter (Boyd, 2012)

The negative effect of birthweight on subsequent performance and the impact that the bottom 20% of pigs have on this period was shown in a study (Schinckel *et al.,* 2004) whereby 433 pigs were followed through from birth to 61 days. Individual pigs were measured at birth, weaning, day 19 post-weaning and day 42 post-weaning. The results showed when pigs at birth were split into five 20 percentile groups the mean weights were 1.14, 1.46, 1.65, 1.88 and 2.28 kg and that the difference in body weights increased with age. At 42 days post-weaning the three heaviest birthweight groups were similar with the second lightest birthweight intermediate and the lightest group being lower. This highlights the negative effect that the bottom 20% of lightweight pigs can have on overall performance and this negative effect would be expected to impact all the way to slaughter (Schinckel and Craig, 2002). The author speculated that the sow's milk production limits the growth of pigs prior to weaning (Le Dividich, 1999) whereby the light birthweight pigs tend to be associated with the posterior teats which produce less milk than the anterior teats. Therefore targeting these lighter pigs by increasing birthweight or putting strategies in place pre- or post-weaning to improve light weight pig performance will be critical in improving overall production performance and reducing live-weight variation.

Work by Leeds University (Isley *et al.,* 2001) showed that birthweight, weaning weight and 20 day post-weaning weight were all important in determining lifetime performance (Table 2). However it was noted that the key opportunities to impact lifetime performance were weaning weight and 20 day post-weaning weight where a 5% improvement could reduce time to market or increase extra gain in the same days to market. Thereby any method of influencing weaning and 20 day post-weaning weight would be advantageous especially in terms of the bottom 20% of the birthweight pigs.

Table 2. Performance improvement to give 1 kg extra at market

Performance parameter	Order of importance	Weight change	% Change	Comment
20 d ADG post-weaning	1	17 g/d	5	Achievable
Weaning weight	2	0.33 kg	5	Achievable
Birthweight	3	0.11 kg	10	Difficult

Note: Adapted from Isley *et al.,* 2001.

Irrespective of genetics the commonality of a greater number of smaller pigs with increasing litter size remains. The bottom 20% of the birthweight pigs are the pigs that are the issue in the production system. Improving the performance of these piglets is critical in optimizing the overall pig unit performance as these pigs have a lower level of survivability and take longer to get to market.

Weaning weight

One common thing that producers understand is the need to maximise weaning weight as a way of improving subsequent post-weaning performance. Although birthweight is an early determinant of lifetime performance, weaning weight is also a key factor (Dunshea *et al.,* 2003 and Douglas *et al.,* 2013). This is well documented with an evaluation in Canada (Wilcock; Unpublished) showing that increasing weaning weight from 3.8 kg to 6 kg improved the 42-day post-weaning performance by 4.2 kg or the equivalent of 45 g/day for a 1 kg improvement in weaning weight. This is supported by work conducted by the Prairie Swine Centre that showed for every 1 kg extra in weaning weight there was an improvement in ADG by 40 g/day through the nursery (Whittington *et al.,* 2005) while Campbell (1990) showed a 35 g/d benefit with a 1 kg weaning weight advantage. This benefit of weaning weight extends to the finishing (Mahan and Lepine, 1991; Wolters and Ellis, 2001 and Cooper *et al.,* 2001) performance with Cooper showing that a 1 kg improvement in weaning translated to 4.2 kg at 20 weeks of age. These trials were focused on performance but more recent commercial research work (Boyd, Personal Communication, 2014) on approximately 800 early weaned pigs showed that increasing weaning weight improved nursery end weight (46 d post-weaning) and finishing (147 d post-weaning) performance as other studies had shown. In early weaned pigs (< 21d) a 1 kg improvement translated into an average 3.4 kg advantage at 147 d post-weaning but more importantly in this study the impact on survivability and top grade pigs was monitored. These results (Figure 4) show the value of weaning weight not just in terms of gain but also in terms of percentage of full value pigs, dead pigs, culled pigs or light pigs whereby increasing weaning weight improved the percentage of full value pigs at the expense of dead, culled and light pigs. The effect of the lightest pigs (3 kg) again is evident with 22% of these pigs dying or being culled before market while in comparison only 9% of the heavy pigs (6 kg) were in this category. This data shows the importance in the producer targeting improved average weaning weights and by doing so it will reduce the number of small pigs at weaning and improve the overall productivity of the unit. Thereby any strategies to improve weaning weight via management or nutrition (sow or piglet) should be considered as a potential way of improving overall unit performance.

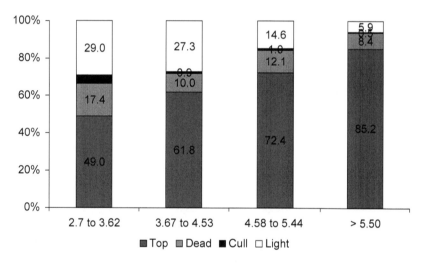

Figure 4. Effect of weaning weight on percentage of top value, dead, cull or light pigs from weaning to market (Personal communication, Boyd, 2014)

20 day post-weaning

Although birth and weaning weights are important in determining lifetime productivity the early post-weaning performance is also critical in not just subsequent gain but improving the number of full value pigs at market. Work at Leeds University (Miller *et al.,* 1999 and Isley 2001) showed that both weaning weight and early post-weaning growth were important on subsequent pig performance. Indeed Miller (1999) showed that there was a strong correlation between both weaning weight and growth rate in week one on subsequent performance post-weaning. Their influence is very similar and also additive.

$$\text{Day 20 Liveweight} = 3.73 + 1.25 \text{ weaning LW} + 8.92 \text{ ADG in week 1}$$
$$(r^2\ 0.798, P < 0.001).$$

This improvement of early nursery performance on lifetime performance has been established by a number of different authors (Tokach *et al.,* 1992; Pluske *et al.,* 1995, 1999, Dunshea *et al.,* 1997; Slade *et al.,* 2000; Kim *et al.,* 2003; Lawlor *et al,* 2002 and Broom *et al.,* 2003) with typically 1 kg out of the nursery equating to 4 days faster to slaughter or an equivalent of an extra 3 to 4 kg of weight in the same days to market.

In contrast the role of compensatory gain based on research trials is again a topic of discussion whereby compensatory gain is described as "irrespective of the pigs early post-weaning performance the weight at slaughter is not significantly different." With this feeding concept it would be possible to lower feed cost in early post-weaning nutrition and still have the same outcome at slaughter thereby minimizing the cost of production. However when reviewed by Wellock *et al.* (2013) it was established that the data was inconsistent especially when compensation was defined as "the ability of restricted pigs exhibiting a significantly faster rate of gain than their non-restricted counterparts in the period of catch up growth in addition to no significant difference in body weight at the end of the catch up period." This was based on well managed research studies and did not even account for the realism of commercial practice whereby sex, genotype, length of sub-optimal nutrition, health and timing as well as the nutrition of the finisher diet needed to enable compensation to have a chance of succeeding would need to be taken into account. With the inconsistent nature of compensatory growth even in a well-controlled research environment (Taylor *et al.,* 2013) the target of getting the pigs off to a better start through appropriate nutrition and management to ensure a fast, economical, growth rate to slaughter should still be the aim to allow for more profitable and sustainable pig production.

Thereby any management or nutritional practices that can be used during this period to increase feed intake and post-weaning performance should be considered. This is a large wide spanning topic (management practices, nutritional concept, compensatory growth) for consideration in this paper so the authors point to the following papers for more specific details (Wilcock, 2009; Wellock *et al.,* 2013; Toplis *et al.,* 2013).

Feeding the pre-weaning piglet to improve weaning weight and lifetime performance

It is recognised that impacting the sow in terms of improving litter weaning weights is a key component of maximising litter weight and that will be discussed later. However are there intervention production strategies that can be used to improve pre-weaning performance directly through the piglet? Two strategies that have been used are creep feeding and milk replacer and the following will highlight some of the benefits and issues these may have in terms of improving weaning and subsequent pig performance.

Creep feeding

Traditionally creep feeding has been associated with later weaned pigs (> 21 days) and was targeted at improving weaning weight. The data in improved weaning weight with the older weaned pig although inconsistent has shown benefits of almost an extra 1 kg in weaning weight (Sprent *et al.*, 2000). Other work however has shown minimal weight improvements of creep feeding on later weaned pigs (Morrison *et al.*, 2008). This may in part be explained by work conducted by Pluske (1995) that showed from a number of trials that the contribution of creep in terms of percent energy intake required to maintain pre-weaning performance was between 1.2 and 17.4%. This suggests that there may be limited opportunity in improving weaning performance but caution must be taken as this data would not be on an individual pig basis. It is believed that creep feeding would be of greater benefit to the smaller pig where intake of creep would likely be higher due to them suckling on the posterior teats which have less milk production. This application however opens up the opportunity of potentially using creep feeds in sows with high litter sizes to improve overall weaning weight. An early weaned piglet study (Klindt, 2003) showed that increasing litter size dropped weaning weight but that with a litter size greater than 8/9 pigs the use of creep feeding, when introduced early, helped improve pre-weaning piglet growth and maintain weaning weight. If however weaning weight improvement is not the only benefit of creep feeding then what are the other potential benefits?

A recent study in Canada (Shea *et al.*, 2013) compared the effect of creep feed in both 21 day and 28 day weaned piglets and found that the creep feeding benefit on weaning weight was consistent irrespective of weaning age with pigs fed creep feed being 0.2 kg heavier. The larger benefit of creep feeding in this case came post-weaning with those pigs eating creep feed having an extra 1.3 kg benefit at the end of nursery regardless of weaning age. The reason for creep feeding has now become more focused on the post-weaning growth benefit as this study showed that the benefits were similar in both early (< 21 days) and later (> 21 days) weaned pigs.

Both European (Bruininx, *et al.*, 2002) and US studies (Sulabo *et al.*, 2010) have shown that using creep feed to increase the number of pigs per litter consuming feed prior to weaning (eaters), results in a better post-weaning performance when compared to pigs that have not consumed creep feed (non-eaters) (Figure 5). In addition it was found that eaters had a significantly greater reduction in pen CV than non-eater pigs at day 28 post-weaning when compared to the same pigs at weaning. It was suggested that individual feed consumption prior to weaning may be an important factor in improving uniformity at the end of the nursery and that this may be attributed to the faster gain in the initial week post-weaning of the smaller pigs. Therefore any nutritional/management practices to stimulate individual pigs to consume creep prior to weaning will potentially benefit post-weaning performance and potentially reduce variation at the end of the nursery.

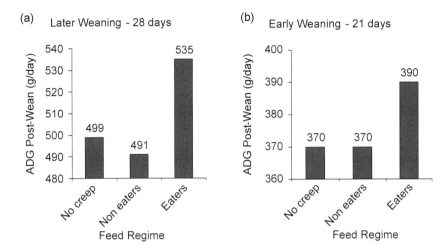

Figure 5. Improving pigs consuming creep feed pre-weaning improves post-weaning average daily gain (a) Bruininx *et al.* (2002); (b) Sulabo *et al.* (2010)

Indeed Sulabo went one step further and found that when a simple creep feed was compared with a complex creep the percentage of eaters within a litter was increased from 28% to 68% with a significant creep feed intake per litter for those litters fed the complex feed ration. This confirmed earlier work by Fraser *et al.* (1994) that also showed increasing creep feed complexity significantly improved pre-weaning feed intake. In addition introducing the creep feed earlier (at day 7 compared to day 14) also improved the number of eaters in the litter by 10% or effectively 1.2 pigs per litter (based on an average 12 pig litter size), (Sulabo *et al.,* 2010). Furthermore, creep feeder type can impact feed intake and percentage of piglets consuming food. Sulabo *et al.* (2010) looked at three types of creep feeders and showed that one particular feeder type (Table 3) increased the percentage of pigs consuming creep by approximately 30% when compared to the other feeders.

Table 3. Creep feeder design on percentage of pigs eating creep

Treatment	Rotary feeder with hopper	Rotary feeder without hopper	Pan feeder	Prob
Creep feeding disappearance (kg)	0.44[a]	1.18[c]	1.24[c]	< 0.1
Proportion of litter eating creep (%)	69.3	47.3	41.6	< 0.1

The benefit that eaters may have over non-eaters when it comes to post-weaning growth is both through improved gut maturity and behavioral response. Bruininx *et al.* (2002) showed that eaters were faster to consume feed post-weaning and had a greater number of visits to the feeders than non-eaters or pigs that did not get creep feed. This combination of quicker to consume feed and more visits to the feeder translates to a greater feed intake and post weaning gain. Pigs that also are fed creep containing complex carbohydrates have also shown improved gastric pepsin and acid production (Cranwell and Stuart, 1984) and enhanced pancreatic and gastric enzymes. This provides the pre-weaning pig with a more mature gut system and may improve the transition through weaning and improve post-weaning growth.

The impact of pre-weaning microflora has been another area of interest in terms of research and the potential application of creep feeds. Australian researchers (Pluske *et al.*, 2005) had found that pigs reared outdoors performed better (greater carcass weight, and dressing weight) than indoor pigs from wean to finish and the question was raised as to whether any substrate effect may be associated with this benefit that could be applied to the creep feed. A subsequent indoor lifetime study showed that the use of an outdoor mix (sow feed, straw, soil and organic matter), when offered as a creep, improved birth to slaughter weight, hot carcass weight and dressing percentage compared to the same pigs offered no creep or a commercial creep. This showed that at least in this specific genetics the use of outdoor material could influence carcass characteristics 20 weeks later. The interest in the difference in microflora depending on if the pigs are born outdoors or indoors is stimulating areas of research to determine if the indoor raised pig can have its microflora changed to that of an outdoor reared pig and if this will impact lifetime performance. A comparison of microflora between pigs, outdoor sow reared, indoor sow reared, and indoor sow isolated with antibiotics saw major differences in the microflora population (Mulder, 2009). The outdoor reared pigs that were exposed to more microbial diversity early on actually showed a lower microbial diversity later on with a high percentage of the beneficial bacteria, *Lactobacillus*. In addition gene expression work showed that there was a higher level of gut immune-stimulation associated with both categories of indoor reared pigs while the outdoor pigs showed a lower level of pro-inflammatory response. This is an area of interest and further development with opportunities to use a creep feed to provide a substrate for the desired microflora in the gut.

With increased pressure on the sow with increasing litter size the use of creep for improving weaning weight, but more importantly post-weaning performance, has stimulated further interest in creep studies.

Recent work in the UK (Almond, Personal Communication, 2013) on creep feeding has shown the benefits a specialist creep can have on nursery and lifetime performance. A series of 6 trials were conducted on late weaned pigs (> 21 days) that showed the use of a specialist creep feed v a standard creep feed from day 4 of age, reduced pre-weaning mortality by 3.2%, increased piglets weaned per litter by 0.4 pigs with an extra weaning weight of 0.28 kg per pig. Subsequent 21 d post-weaning performance was also improved on pigs fed the specialist creep feed with pigs showing an average improvement of 0.78 kg of extra gain. It was also found where individual pigs were measured that the use of the specialist creep feed decreased body weight variation at nursery exit (Figure 6).

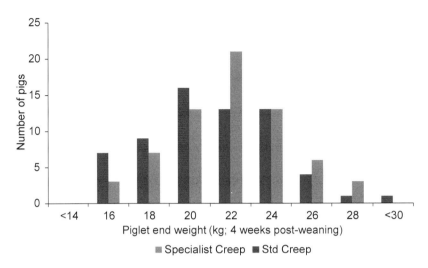

Figure 6. Impact of creep feeding on variation in pig weight at 28 days post-weaning (Personal Communication: Almond, 2013)

One of the aforementioned studies was conducted at Harper Adams University. In this study pigs were fed a standard creep or specialised creep pre-weaning after which all pigs were fed a common feeding regime to slaughter. The results showed that pigs that had been fed the specialist creep pre-weaning had an extra 4.3 kg at slaughter (Figure 7). This series of studies confirm the importance that creep feeding can have on pre-weaning and lifetime performance whereby the percentage of small pigs are reduced and that different creep feeds can impact performance differently.

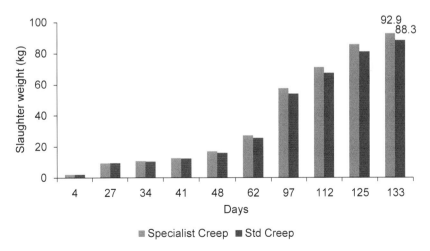

Figure 7. The effect of feeding a specialist creep on lifetime performance. (Creep was fed until weaning at 27 d after which all pigs were fed the same feed programme) (Personal Communication: Almond, 2013)

Milk replacer

The use of milk replacer to improve weaning weight and sow efficiency is not a new concept and in 1993, research (Harrell *et al.*, 1993) showed that after 10 days pigs were limited in terms of gain when on the sow compared to pigs artificially reared. In addition the same researchers demonstrated that artificially reared pigs grew faster (395 v 232 g/d) from birth to weaning (21 days) when compared to sow reared pigs.

A quick review of the literature shows the effectiveness of supplemental milk replacer in improving pre-weaning performance (Table 4) with an average 19% improvement in growth compared to sow reared pigs.

Table 4 Effect of milk replacer on pre-weaning growth rate

		MR length	Lactation length	Pre-weaning growth rate	% Diff.	Reference
Trial 1a	No MR		21	222		Azain *et al.*, 1996
Winter	MR	21	21	247	+11.2	
Trial 1b	No MR		21	166		
Summer	MR	21	21	224	+34.9%	
Trial 2	No MR		28	238		King *et al.*, 1998
	MR	24	28	297	+24.7%	
Trial 3	No MR		20	223		Dunshea *et al.*, 1997
	MR	10	20	291	+30%	
Trial 4	No MR		28	214		Campbell *et al.*, 1990
	MR	10	28	264	+23.3%	
Trial 5	No MR		21	192		Wolters *et al.*, 2002
	MR	18	21	236	+22.9%	
Trial 6a	No MR - Gilt	23	26	219		Miller *et al.*, 2012
Winter	MR - Gilt	23	26	233	+6.3%	
	No MR - Sow	23	26	230		
	MR - Sow	23	26	245	+6.5%	
Trial 6b	No MR - Gilt	23	26	209		
Summer	MR- Gilt	23	26	240	+14.8%	
	No MR - Sow	23	26	200		
	MR - Sow	23	26	230	+15.0%	
Average Improvement					+18.96	

The use of supplemental milk replacer has been therefore proposed as a management tool to improve weaning weight and reduce mortality of the pigs especially the bottom 20% of birth weight pigs associated with large litter size. Supplemental milk replacer is often supplied via cups that are added into the crate so that piglets have easy access. This cup is plumbed into a tank that contains the mixed milk replacer and allows a constant supply to the cups as the pigs consume the milk replacer. When using this system with early weaned pigs (< 21 days), internal research (unpublished) showed that the use of supplemental milk replacer reduced the percentage of light pigs (< 5 kg) from 22% to 10% of the total pigs weaned and reduced the overall variation in the litters at weaning. Further work (Wellock, personal communication), showed that in high litter size (> 13 pigs born alive) the effect of supplementing milk replacer improved weaning weight by 0.33 kg (7.56kg v 7.89 kg) and reduced mortality by 3.7% resulting in an extra 0.5 pig weaned per litter (11.3 v 11.8 piglets weaned). This would support the work of Wolter *et al.* (2002), where the results of using milk replacer not only improved weaning weight but also suggested a reduction in pre-weaning mortality.

In specific circumstances the use of milk replacer as the sole source of nutrient supply in pigs weaned at 2 days (Cabrera *et al.*, 2002) of age has been accessed. The results showed that it was possible to wean pigs at 2 days onto a milk replacer with a reduction in pre-weaning mortality and improved performance of the small birth-weight piglet. This improvement was back to a pre-weaning performance level typically seen with average birthweight pigs This practice is now often used with rescue decks where the smallest pigs from a room of sows are separated from the sows after 48 hours (to allow for colostrum intake) and placed (max 12 pigs per crate) into the deck situated normally above the farrowing pens. Milk replacer is then fed to these pigs via cups in the crate and typically after 4 days dry feed is also introduced. This not only improves the small pig performance but also provides more teat space for those piglets remaining on the sow. This improves average weaning weight but also pre-weaning mortality ensuring more pigs are weaned per sow per year.

Although the data on supplemental and full replacement of milk replacer supports improvements in pre-weaning mortality and weaning weight the impact on the subsequent lifetime performance is mixed. Researchers have (Wolters *et al.*, 2002; Miller *et al.*, 2012) showed that pigs fed supplemental milk replacer pre-weaning did not improve gain from weaning to slaughter compared to traditionally reared piglets. Contrary to this Dunshea (1999) and Spencer (2003) showed that the use of supplemental milk replacer pre-weaning improved post-weaning performance.

As a tool, milk replacer could be used to improve the mean weaning weights as well as reducing both pre-weaning mortality and weaning weight variation. Each production system is specific and it is vital to target milk replacer technology to specific piglets and management practices to achieve improvements in survivability and weight gain of selected piglets with non-impaired growth competencies. Proper application of milk replacer can increase mean weights and reduce total litter variance.

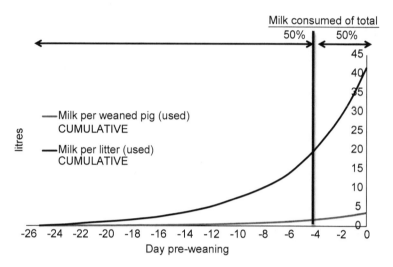

Figure 8. Milk consumed per weaned piglet or weaned litter(Approximately 50% of milk replacer is consumed in last 4 days before weaning)(Weaning Age – 26 days)(Personal Communication: Wellock, 2013)

Milk replacer typically should be used with large litter sizes (> 12 pigs born alive). Notice should however be taken of the extra management time and costs associated with the use of milk replacer. For example in the use of supplementary milk replacer it has been shown to be more cost effective to use milk replacer up to 4 days pre-weaning and then switch off the access to milk replacer. This practice saves almost 50% of the milk replacer consumption (Figure 8) that would be consumed to weaning, thereby 50% of the cost, while not negatively impacting the benefit milk replacer has on pre-weaning performance.

Sow nutrition – improving weaning weight

Lactating sow nutrient intake

The obvious key to improve weaning weight is by targeting increased feed intake and water intake by the lactation sow especially in summer when intakes traditionally drop. The following is just a brief review of some of the key points of stimulating feed intake and the authors point to Vignola, 2009 and Neill and Williams, 2010 for more in-depth review on sow production.

To optimise lactation intake it is necessary to ensure that pregnant sows are not overfed and over conditioned; ideally they should be in the 3 to 3.5 range on a scale of 1 to 5. Prior to farrowing, feed intake should be dropped to approximately 2 kg to ensure early lactation feed intake is maximised and thereby minimising health issues in lactation. Feed intake will not be maximised without sufficient water intake and so sows should have access to fresh water with good flow (2 litres per minute for a bite drinker) or even liquid or wet feeding to stimulate intake. Feed intake has also been stimulated by two management practices; the introduction of self-feeders has stimulated lactation feed intake over the traditional hand feeding system by 7% while the use of low level increment of feed intake in the first 4 days post-farrow (1.8 kg, 1.8kg 2.7 kg and 2.7 kg respectively) before going to *ad libitum* feeding has helped stimulate overall lactation feed intake (Neill and Williams. 2010). The impact of temperature is important in lactating sows as with an increased level of feed intake the sows' temperature requirement drops and so if the room is too warm the sows will lower feed intake. It is therefore important to target the sows' thermal neutral zone (between 12 to 20° C) to maximise intake while Vignola (2009) noted that for every degree above 20° C there is a reduction in feed intake of approximately 0.15 kg per day. Most units tend to typically target 18 to 20 ° C. Obviously this is the reason for sow intake drop during summer when room temperatures are difficult to control and different genetic lines will likely be affected differently. Farrowing room hygiene plays an important role in feed intake especially in wet feeding were it is important to not let feed go stale and moldy. The importance of focusing on high intake coupled with a high nutrient dense diet will maximise the nutrient intake to the sow, increasing milk production and improving weaning weights.

If we can stimulate feed intake as the number one target are there any other areas that can be targeted to improve weaning weight outside of the nutrient specification of the diet? The following looks at three feed ingredients that are commonly used in lactation in the market and are generally targeted at improving average weaning weight with a high number of pigs weaned per sow. Any opportunity to improve the average weaning weight will improve the performance opportunity of the bottom 20% of pigs.

Live yeast

Live yeast is a probiotic and has been used extensively in the dairy market to improve dry matter intake and increase milk production. A key mechanism is the ability for the live yeast to scavenge oxygen and provide the correct environment for beneficial bacteria such as fibre degrading bacteria to grow. This thereby improves nutrient utilisation and milk production.

In the pig, use of live yeast has mainly been focused in more of the stressful periods of pork production such as lactation and nursery pigs. The use of a live yeast in lactation has shown benefits in terms of weaning weight improvement and pre-weaning mortality (Supple *et al.*, 2012). A series of six internal research and commercial studies support this data with the use of a live yeast in lactation improving weaning weights by an average of 7.95% and reducing pre-weaning mortality by an average of 2.73% (for example 15% to 12.23%). The mechanism that a live yeast acts within the sow is still uncertain but it is thought a combination of improving the gut environment, improving hind gut fermentation and energy utilisation, binding of pathogenic bacteria (Trckova *et al.*, 2014) as well as supporting the immune system translate into better nutrient utilisation by the sow. This improved nutrient utilisation improves the milk nutrient density and thereby improves pre-weaning piglet growth. Live yeast also improves feed intake by 3 to 4% (Internal Research) which can be important especially in summer months when intake traditionally drops. Live yeast also can improve the level of immunoglobulins in the colostrum and milk (Jurgens, 1997; Jang *et al.*, 2012) which can improve piglet immunity during the pre-weaning and post-weaning period thereby reducing pre-weaning mortality.

Carnitine

Carnitine can be synthesised by the body from protein bound lysine and methionine and so does not need to be an essential component of the diet. However in the young neonate the ability to synthisise carnitine is limited and so supplementing the early weaned pig with carnitine may be beneficial in terms of pre-weaning performance. L-carnitine is essential in the transportation of long and medium chain fatty acids across the mitrochondrial membrane for B-oxidation and therefore low levels of carnitine may lead to suboptimal usage of fatty acids. As sows' colostrum and milk is a readily available source of carnitine it was thought that the use of carnitine in sow diets may improve weaning weight. The use of carnitine in both dry and lactating sows is well documented and a quick review of the literature shows that in the following studies (Musser *et al.*, 1999; Eder *et al.*, 2001 and Ramanau *et al.*, 2002, 2004 and 2008) the use of carnitine in dry and lactating sows improves birth and weaning weights. Based on these studies weaning weights were improved by an average of 0.55 kg per pig. In one study (Ramanau *et al.*, 2004) the use of carnitine in dry and lactation showed that the nutrient content of sows' milk did not change with the exception that the carnitine supplemented sows showed a higher level of milk carnitine. However the level of nutrient intake into the piglets was increased as the carnitine supplemented sows showed a higher level of milk production.

Bacillus species

The use of *bacillus* species as probiotics is well established in post-weaning pigs with good evidence of improved performance. However the use of *bacillus* in the sow is a more recent application and similar to live yeast it acts as a probiotic whereby it improves nutrient utilisation resulting in improved milk protein and milk fat (Jorgensen, 2005). This was linked in this study to improved weaning weight (0.38 kg) and reduced pre-weaning mortality (5.1%) while those sows fed the probiotic had less weight loss at weaning. Other studies (Zerrahn *et al.*, 2008; Lilija *et al.*, 2012; Baker *et al.*, 2013) have shown benefit in pre-weaning mortality from a negative effect of 1.1% to a positive effect of 3.9%. The full mechanism behind the *bacillus* species is uncertain but it is believed that when in the gastrointestinal tract it consumes oxygen as well as producing enzymes. This provides a positive environment for *lactobacilli* and these compete with pathogenic bacteria improving gut health and nutrient utilisation.

Feeding the post-weaning pig

The benefit of improving 20 day and nursery post-weaning growth on lifetime performance and improving the bottom 20% of the light pigs has already been discussed. Improving performance can be a result of many different factors such as management, nutrition or environmental. However this section will look at two areas covering management of the feed program for small pigs and the use of low phytate nutrition to improve post-weaning performance.

Feeding programme

Starter regimes are critical to maximise pig performance during the nursery phase as pigs transition from liquid to solid feed. However it may be necessary to feed pigs differently depending on their birth and weaning weight in order to improve the small pig performance post-weaning. A recent study (Douglas *et al.*, 2014) looked at the effect that feeding a high specification, high digestible feed program can have on small pig performance.

At birth pigs were classified into light birth weight (LBW) pigs (< 1.25 kg) or normal birth weight (NBW) pigs (> 1.25 kg). Pigs were then weaned at 28 days and allocated to one of six treatments, with 4 treatments on LBW and 2 treatments on NBW pigs. The 4 treatments on LBW were fed a high (H) or standard (S) starter feed regime (Table 5). After the starter feed allocation H and S treated pigs were then fed a standard link feed or an increased level (extra 2.5 kg) of link feed. The NBW pigs were fed the high or standard starter feed regime with no additional link feed. After the link feed all pigs were fed a common weaner feed.

The results confirmed that birth weight was as expected correlated to weaning weight and that when the LBW pigs were fed the same standard post-weaning program as the NBW pigs (A and B v E and F) the NBW pigs were significantly (P < 0.001) heavier (30.6 kg v 27.4 kg) at day 70 and consumed more feed (P < 0.02). Within the LBW the best performing pigs were those that were fed the high specification (B and D) starter feed as they had a significantly improved gain at day 70 over the standard (A and C) starter program (29.0 kg v 27.3 kg). In addition those LBW pigs that were fed (C and D) extra link feed also improved nursery exit weights compared to pigs fed no (A and B) extra link (28.9 v 27.4 kg). The best performing LBW pigs were those fed the high specification starter feed and extra link feed (D) and when these were compared to the NBW (E and F) pigs it was shown that at day 70 the LBW pigs were not significantly different to the NBW pigs (30.1 kg v 30.6 kg). More importantly not only was the LBW pig performance (D) improved by the high spec, extra link feeding regime but it was at a similar cost/kg of gain as all LBW pigs and returned the greatest margin over feed.

Table 5 Effect of post-weaning feed programme on light and normal birthweight pigs

| | | | Birthweight | | | | |
| | | | Lights (LBW) | | | Normal (NBW) | |
Treatment		A	B	C	D	E	F
Birth Weight (kg)		1.05	1.10	1.06	1.09	1.82	1.81
Wean weight (Day 28) (kg)		7.15	7.14	7.26	6.85	8.67	8.57
FEEDING REGIME	Lysine %						
Diet A (kg/d)	1.75	-	2.5	-	2.5	-	2.5
Diet B (kg/d)	1.60	2	2	2	2	2	2
Diet C (kg/d)	1.50	3	3	5.5	5.5	3	3
Weaner (kg/d)	1.40	26.6	21.6	22.1	20.6	30.9	27.6
Total starter (kg/d) [Diet A + B + C]		5	7.5	7.5	10	5	7.5
Total feed (kg/d)		31.6	29.1	29.6	30.6	35.9	35.1
PERFORMANCE							
Day 70 weight (kg)		26.9	27.9	27.7	30.1	30.9	30.3
ADG d 28-70 (kg/d)		0.470	0.494	0.487	0.554	0.529	0.517
ADFI d 28-70 (kg/d)		0.752	0.693	0.705	0.729	0.855	0.836
FCR d 28-70		1.60	1.40	1.45	1.32	1.61	1.62
ECONOMICS							
Total feed cost (£/pig)		13.06	13.93	12.91	15.04	14.60	16.09
Cost/kg gain (£)		0.66	0.67	0.63	0.65	0.66	0.74
Return Over Feed @ £1.70/kg DW		12.13	12.54	13.16	14.61	13.74	11.62

This data clearly shows that the performance of small pigs at birth can be influenced by the post-weaning feeding program. Increasing the feed level of a higher specification starter feed while feeding more link feed can improve the performance of the light birth weight up to that of the normal birth weight pig by nursery exit. This improved performance was achieved while delivering an extra margin over feed showing that this may be a cost effective solution to improve small pig performance. This data is supported by earlier work (Morrison *et al.*, 2007 and Beaulieu *et al.*, 2010) suggesting that the strategic use of high quality, high specification diets may be a management tool to improve the performance of light weight pigs to that seen with the average weight pig. This could be a cost effective solution (greater margin over feed) to improving light weight pig performance.

Low phytate nutrition – starter feed

Traditionally the use of phytase in starter feed has been limited as Auspurger *et al.* (2004) showed that P release from phytase was reduced in the presence of pharmacological levels of zinc. However this was with an older generation phytase and at standard levels of inclusion targeting P release. Recent work in piglets however has looked at the use of superdose (> 2000 FTU/kg) levels of phytase to break down phytate as an anti-nutrient in starter feeds containing pharmacological zinc levels to improve performance.

It has been known for some time that phytate is an anti-nutrient in terms of reducing mineral bioavailability but in recent years there has been research confirming the negative impact of phytate on amino acid, protein, trace mineral, calcium, sodium and energy utilisation by the animal. This area is too detailed to cover in this paper, and the reader is pointed to Cowieson *et al.* (2009, 2011) for more information.

It is thought that phytate, when soluble (low pH), may bind proteins through electrostatic charges making protein refractory to pepsin digestion. Alternatively phytate may compete with proteins and other compounds for water. Regardless of the mechanism, the reduced protein solubility results in an increased production of HCl, pepsin, mucin, bile and bicarbonate in the stomach and duodenum by the animal. This results in an increased maintenance energy requirement, endogenous amino acid loss and sodium flow into the lumen, with the latter negatively impacting active nutrient transport.

This negative impact on protein solubility effect not just vegetable sources such as corn and soybean meal but also non-vegetable proteins, with casein being an example. This latter example is important when considering complex piglet starter feeds which traditionally have lower vegetable protein and more animal and milk proteins. This high use of animal/milk proteins at the expense of vegetable proteins reduces the level of dietary phytate and it is often thought that this may minimise the negative impact of phytate. However, small changes in the phytate concentration of the diet can significantly impact growth performance. For example, increasing the dietary phytate concentration by only 0.16% can reduce ADG by 3% and feed efficiency by 7%, particularly in piglets seven to 14 days post-weaning (Walk *et al.*, 2014). This slight increase in dietary phytate could be the result of a 2 to 5% increase in the inclusion of high phytate grains, such as full fat rice bran or soybean meal, or the result of natural variation of the phytate concentration of grains. For example, the phytate concentration in commonly used feed ingredients such as corn, wheat or soybean meal can range by 10 to 30% from average values. Therefore, even small incremental changes of dietary phytate can have a significant impact on piglet growth performance.

Through phytase superdosing it is possible to minimise the anti-nutrient effect of phytate and improve energy, amino acid and mineral utilisation thereby eliciting a response in the newly weaned pig. A secondary more recent explanation of the benefit of superdosing phytase has been linked to the production of inositol. Inositol plays a role in many metabolic functions within the animal including lipid and phospholipid metabolism, secondary messengers and re-phosphorylation within the cell to phytate which is known to be an antioxidant. Inositol has been shown to improve animal performance (Zyla et al., 2004) while Bedford et al. (2013), showed that the inositol production from superdosing phytase may account for 30% of the superdosing response. Further work in pigs (Wilcock et al., 2014) and broilers (Walk et al., 2013) showed that there was a positive correlation between increasing the dietary dose of a modified E. Coli phytase with increased inositol measured in the stomach/gizzard of the animal and improvement in gain and feed conversion.

A series of studies have been conducted (Walk et al., 2012; Cordero et al., 2013; Bradley et al., 2014; Walk et al., 2014; Walk et al., 2014 and Wellock et al., 2014) looking at the impact that high levels (> 2000 FTU/kg) of a modified E. Coli phytase can have on post-weaning pig performance in diets with pharmacological levels of zinc. In these studies the phytase was added over the top of a starter feed diet designed to meet the pigs' requirement for phosphorus and calcium. The outcome of these studies showed that the use of superdosing phytase from weaning to 21 days post-weaning improved ADG by 7.2% and FCR by 4.2%. As all diets were designed to meet the requirements of the animal this data suggests that the response to the superdosing phytase was associated with phytate breakdown and not phosphorus provision.

This new application of using superdosing levels of phytase in starter feeds that contain pharmacological levels of zinc to breakdown phytate as an anti-nutrient could potentially be used to improve post-weaning performance and minimise the impact of the small pig effect.

Conclusion

The current pig market continues to target an increased litter size thereby maximising the amount of pork output per annum at a lower cost base. However with the hyper-prolific sows there is a concern that intrauterine crowding is having a negative impact on birthweight and subsequent performance. This has led to greater litter sizes and a higher percentage of smaller pigs to manage and it is these pigs that are the issue in the production system with higher mortalities/morbidity and less full value pigs going to market. Moving forward there are strategies that can be used to improve the small pig effect such as the pre-weaning use of specialist creep feeding and the use of milk replacer, the post-weaning use of different feeding programs and new applications of enzymes. These pre-weaning applications may take up more labour and management time but the performance benefits may be warranted. In addition a greater focus on the sow in terms of selecting for increased uterine capacity may be advantageous as well as ensuring the lactating sow is managed and fed correctly to maximise milk production.

Acknowledgements

The authors would like to thank Dean Boyd at Hanor Company, USA and Kayleigh Almond at Primary Diets, UK for sharing internal research data for use in this review.

References

Augspurger, N. R., and Baker, D.H. (2004) High dietary phytase levels maximize phytate-phosphorus utilization but do not affect protein utilization in chicks fed phosphorus or amino acid-deficient diets. *Journal of Animal Science*, **82**, 1100–1107.

Azain, J.J., Tomkins, T., Sowinski, J.S., Arentson, R.A., and Jewell, D.E. (1996) Effect of supplemental pig milk replacer on litter performance: Seasonal variation in response. *Journal of Animal Science*, **74**, 2095-2202.

Baker, A.A, Davis, E., Spencer, J.D., Moser, R. and Rehberger, T. (2013) The effect of Bacillus-based direct fed microbial supplemented to sows on the gastrointestinal microbiota of their neonatal piglets. *Journal of Animal Science*, **91**, 3390-3399.

Beaulieu, A.D., Aalhus, J.L., Williams, N.H. and Patience, J.F. (2010), Impact of piglet birthweight, birth order, and litter size on subsequent growth performance , carcass quality, muscle composition and eating quality of pork. *Journal of Animal Science*, **88**, 2767-2778.

Bedford, M.R. and Rama Rao, S.V. (2013) Effects of inositol or phytase alone in combination, in diets deficient, adequate or in excess of dietary phosphate. *Poultry Science Annual Meeting*, San Diego, US, Abstract 110.

Berard, J., Pardo, C.E., Bethaz, S., Kreuzer, M. and Bee, G. (2010) Intrauterine crowding decreases average birth weight and affects muscle fiber hyperplasia in piglets. *Journal of Animal Science*, **88**, 3242-3250.

Boyd, R.D. (2012) Integrating science into practice and getting it right, Howard Dunne Memorial Lecture, *43rd Annual American Association of Swine Practitioners Conference*, Colorado, Denver, US.

Bradley, C.L., Walk, C.L., Cordero, G. and Wilcock, P. (2014) Pharmacological ZnO dose and superdoses of phytase on piglet growth performance and cost of gain from d 0 to 21 post-weaning. *Animal Society of Animal Science - Midwest Meetings*, Des Moines, IA, US, Abstract 141.

Broom, L. J., Miller, H.M., Kerr, K.J. and Toplis, P. (2003) Removal of both zinc oxide and avilamycin from the post-weaning diet: consequences for performance through to slaughter, *Animal. Science*, **77**, 79-84.

Bruininx, E.M.A, Binnendijk, G.P., van der Peet-Schwering, C.M.C., Scharma, J.W., den Hartog, L.A., Everts, H. and Beynen, A.C. (2002) Effect of creep feed consumption on individual feed intake characteristics and performance of group-housed weanling pigs. *Journal of Animal Science*, **80**, 1413-1418.

Cabrera, R., Boyd, R.D. and Vignes, J. (2003) Management of early-weaned (2-d), artificially-reared low birth-weight pigs. In *North Carolina Pig Nutrition Conference, Raleigh, NC, USA.*

Campbell, R.G. (1990) The nutrition and management of pigs to 20 kg liveweight. In *Pig Rations Assessment and Formulation, Proceedings of the Refresher Course for Veterinarians.* University of Sydney, Australia pp 123-126.

Cooper, D.R., Patience, J.F., Gonyou, H.W. and Zijlstra R.T. (2001) Characterization of within pen and within room variation in pigs from birth to market: variation in birthweight and days to market. In *Monograph 01-03. Prairie Swine Centre Inc.*, Saskatoon, SK.

Cordero, G., Santos, T., Walk. C. L. and Wilcock, P. (2013) Inclusion of high levels of phytase (Quantum Blue) improves the performance of pigs from weaning to 21 days post-weaning *Animal Society of Animal Science - Midwest Meetings*, Des Moines, IA, US Abstract P097.

Cowieson, A.J., Bedford, M.R., Selle, P. H. and Ravindran, V. (2009) Phytate and microbial phytase; implications for endogenous nitrogen losses and nutrient availability. *World Poultry Science Journal*, **65**, 401-418.

Cowieson, A.J., Wilcock, P. and Bedford, M.R. (2011) Superdosing effects of phytase in poultry and other monogastrics. *World Poultry Science Journal*, **65**, 401-418.

Cranwell, P.D. and Stuart, S.J. (1984) The effect of diet and liveweight on gastric secretion in the young pig. *Proceedings of the Australian Society of Animal Production*, **15**, 669.

Douglas, S.L., Edwards, S.A., Sutcliffe, E., Knap, P.W. and Kyriazakis, I. (2013) Identification of risk factors associated with poor lifetime growth performance in pigs. *Journal of Animal Science*, **91**, 4123-4132.

Douglas, S.L., Wellock, I., Edwards, S.A. and Kyriazakis, I. (2014) High specification diets improve the performance of low birth weights to 10 weeks of age. *Journal of Animal Science,* In Press.

Dunshea, F.R., Eason, P.J., Kerton, D.J. Morrish, L., Cox, L.H. and King, R.H. (1997) Supplemental milk around weaning can increase live weight at slaughter. In *Manipulating Pig Production VI, Australian Pig Science Association*, Werribee, pp68-69. Edited by P.D. Cranwell.

Dunshea, F. R., Kerton, D.J., Eason, P.J. and King, R. H. (1999) Supplemental skim milk before and after weaning improves growth performance of pigs. *Australian Journal of Agricultural Research*, **50**, 1165–1170.

Dunshea, F.R., Kerton, D.K., Cranwell, P.D. , Campbell, R.G., Mullan, B.P., King, R.H., Power, G.N. and Pluske, J.R. (2003) Lifetime and post-weaning determinants of performance indices of pigs, Australian Journal of Agricultural Research, **54**, 363-370.

Fix, J. and See, T. (2009) Piglet birth weight affects future growth, composition and mortality. *Swine*

News, North Carolina State Swine Extension, **32**, No. 2.

Foxcroft, G.R., Dixon, W.T., Novak, S., Putman, C.T., Town, S.C. and Vinsky, M.D.A. (2006) The biological basis for prenatal programing of postnatal performance in pigs. *Journal of Animal Science*, **84**, E105-E112.

Fraser, D, Feddes, J.R.R. and Pajor, E.A. (1994) The relationship between creep feeding behaviour of piglets and adaption to weaning: Effect of diet quality. *Canadian Journal of Animal Science*, **74**, 1-6.

Harrell, R.J., Thomas, M.J. and Boyd, R.D. (1993) Limitations of sow milk yield on baby pig growth. In *Proceedings of 1993 Cornell Nutrition Conference for Feed Manufacturers*. Cornell University, Ithaca, NY, pp 156-164.

Isley, S.E., Broom L.J. and Miller H.M. (2001) Birth weight and weaning weight as predictors of pig weight at slaughter. In *Manipulating pig production VIII, Australian Pig Science Association*, Werribee, Victoria 3030, Australia. Edited by P.D. Cranwell.

Jang, Y.D., Kang, K.W., Piao, L.J., Jeong, T.S., Auclair, E., Jonvel, S., D'Inca, R. and Kim, Y.Y. (2013) Effects of live yeast supplementation to gestation and lactation diets on reproductive performance, immunological parameters and milk composition in sows. *Livestock Science*, **152**, 167-173.

Jurgens, M. H., Rikabi, R. A. and Zimmerman., R.D. (1997). The effects of dietary active dry yeast supplement on performance of sows during gestation-lactation and their pigs. *Journal of Animal. Science*, **75**, 593-597.

Jorgensen, J.N. (2005) Probiotics improve sow and litter performance. International Pig Topics, **20**, 11-13.

Kim, J.H., Heo, K.N., Odle, J., Han, I.H. and Harrell, R.J. (2001) Liquid diets accelerate the growth of easily weaned pigs and the effects are maintained to market weight, *Journal of Animal Science*, **79**, 427-434.

King, R.H., Boyce, J.M. and Dunshea, E.R. (1998) The effect of supplemental nutrients on the growth performance of suckling pigs. *Australian Journal of Agricultural Science*, **49**, 1-5.

Klindt, J. (2003) Influence of litter size and creep feeding on pre-weaning gain and influence of pre-weaning growth on growth to slaughter in barrows. *Journal of Animal Science*, **81**, 2434-2439.

Lawlor, P.G., Lynch, P.B., Caffrey, P.J. and O'Doherty, J.V. (2002) Effect of pre– and post–weaning management on subsequent pig performance to slaughter and carcass quality, *Animal. Science*, **75**, 245-256.

Le Dividich, J. (1999) A Review- Neonatal and weaner pig: Management to reduce variation. In *Manipulating pig production VII, Australian Pig Science Association*, Werribee, Victoria 3030, Australia pp 135. Edited by P.D. Cranwell.

Lilija, D. and Sanita, B. (2012) Probiotic Bioplus 2B effect on sows productivity and piglet weight. *Seria Zootehnie*, **57**, 266-269.

Mahan, D.C. and Lepine, A.J. (1991) The effect of pig weaning weight and associated nursery feeding programme on subsequent performance to 105 kg. *Journal of Animal Science*, **66**, 1370-1378.

Miller, H.M., Toplis P. and Slade. R.D. (1999) Weaning weight and daily live-weight gain in the week after weaning predict piglet performance. In *(P.D Cranwell, Ed.)Manipulating pig production VII, Australian Pig Science Association*, Werribee, Victoria 3030, Australia. pp

130 – 130. Edited by P.D. Cranwell.

Miller, Y.J., Collins, A,M., Smits, R.J., Thomson, P.C. and Holyoake, P.K. (2012) Providing supplemental milk to piglets pre-weaning improves the growth but not survival of gilt progeny compared with sow progeny. *Journal of Animal Science*, **90**, 5078-5085.

Morrison, R., Pluske, J. Smits, R., Henman, D. and Collins, C. (2008) Creep feeding, weaning age interactions with creep feeding. In *Feed Intake Innovations, Cooperative Research Centre, Section 2B, Report 3-3*, Australia.

Morrison, R., Pluske, J. Smits, R., Henman, D. and Collins, C. (2009) The use of high cost weaner diets to improve post-weaning growth performance. In *Feed Intake Innovations, Cooperative Research Centre Section 2B, Report 3*, Australia.

Mulder, I.E., Schmidt, B., Stokes, C. R., Lewis, M., Bailey, Mick., Aminov, R.I., Prosser, J.I., Gill, B.P., Pluske, J.R., Mayer, C., Musk, C.C. and Kelly, D. (2009) Environmentally-acquired bacteria influence microbial diversity and natural innate immune responses at gut surfaces. *BMC Biology,* **7,** 79-99.

Musser., R.E., Goodband, R.D., Tokach, M.D. and Owen K.Q., Nelson, J.L., Blum, S.A., Campbell, R.G., Smits, R., Dritz, S.S. and Civis, C.A. (1999) Effects of L-carnitine fed during gestation and lactation on sow and litter performance. *Journal of Animal Science*, 77, 3289-3295.

Neill, C. and Williams, N. (2011) Milk production and nutrient requirements of the modern sow. In *Proceedings of the 10th London Swine Conference*, London, Ontario, pp 23-33. Edited by J.M. Murphy.

PigCHAMP (2005-2012) Benchmarking Country Summaries, 2005 to 2012, *www. PigCHAMP. com*, PigCHAMP Inc. Ames Iowa.

Pluske, J.R., Williams, I. H. and Aherne, F.X. (1995) Nutrition of the neonatal pig. In *The neonatal pig development and survival.* Cab International. Wallingford, UK. pp. 187-235. Edited by M.A. Varley.

Pluske, J.R., Pearson, G., Morel, P.C.H, King, M. H., Skilton, G. and Skilton, R. (1999). A bovine colostrum product in the weaner diet increases growth and reduces days to slaughter. In *Manipulating Pig Production VII, Australian Pig Science Association*, Werribee. pp 256. Edited by M.A. Varley.

Pluske, J.R., Payne, H.G. Williams, I.H. and Mullan, B.P. (2005) Early feeding for lifetime performance of pigs. *Recent Advances in Animal Nutrition in Australia*, **15**, 171-181.

Ramanu, A., Kluge, H., Spilke, J. and Eder, K. (2002) Reproductive performance of sows supplemented with dietary L-carnitine over three reproductive cycles. *Archive Animal Nutrition*, **56**, 287-296.

Ramanu A., Kluge, H., Spilke, J. and Eder, K. (2004) Supplementation of sows with L-carnitine during pregnancy and lactation improves the growth of piglets during the suckling period through increased milk production. *Journal of Nutrition*, **134**, 86-92.

Ramanau, A., Kluge, H., Spilke, J. and Eder, K. (2008) Effects of dietary supplementation of L-carnitine on the reproductive performance of sows in production stocks. *Livestock. Science*, **113**, 34–42.

Schinckel, A.P. and Craig, B.A. (2002) Evaluation of alternative nonlinear mixed effects models of swine growth. *The Professional Animal Scientist*, **18**, 219-226.

Schinckel, A.P., Pas, J., Ferrel, J., Einstein, M.E., Pearce, S.M. and Boyd, R.D. (2004) Analysis of pig growth from birth to sixty days of age. *The Professional Animal Scientist*, **20**, 79-86.

Shea, J., Gillis, A., Brown, J. and Beaulieu, A.D. (2013) Creep feeding in the farrowing room, do outcomes depend on the weaning age? In *Prairie Swine Centre Annual Report 2012-2013*, Saskatchewan, Canada. pp 36-37.

Slade, R.D. and Miller, H.M. (2000) Early post-weaning benefits of porcine plasma remerge in later growth performance. In: *Proceedings of the British Society of Animal Science Winter Meeting 2000*, pp 120.

Spencer, J. D., Boyd, R.D., Cabrera, R. and Allee, G. L. (2003) Early weaning to reduce tissue mobilization in lactating sows and milk supplementation to enhance pig weaning weight during extreme heat stress. *Journal of Animal Science*, **81**, 2041–2052.

Sprent, M., Cole, M.A. and Varley, M.A. (2000) The use of supplementary creep feed for pre-weaned piglets on subsequent performance. *Proceedings of British Society of Animal Science Occasional Meetings- The Weaner Pig*. University of Nottingham, Nottingham, UK.

Sulabo, R.C., Jacela, J.Y., Tokach, M.D., Dritz, S.S., Goodband, R.D., DeRouchery, J.M. and Nelssen, J.L. (2010) Effects of lactation feed intake and creep feeding on sow and piglet performance. *Journal of Animal Science*, **88**, 3145-3153.

Sulabo, R.C., Tokach, M.D., Dritz, S.S., Goodband, R.D., DeRouchery, J.M. and Nelssen, J.L. (2010) Effects of varying creep feeding duration on the proportion of pigs consuming creep feed and neonatal pig performance. *Journal of Animal Science*, **88**, 3154-3162.

Sulabo, R.C., Tokach, M.D., Dritz, S.S., Goodband, R.D., DeRouchery, J.M. and Nelssen, J.L. (2010) Effects of creep feeder design and feed accessibility on pre-weaning pig performance and the proportion of pigs consuming creep feed. *Journal of Swine Health and Production*, **18**, 174–181.

Supple, A., Rosener, D. and Chevaux, E. (2012) Live yeast supplementation to periparturient sows during the summer. *Allen D Leman Swine Conference*, Minneapolis, Minnesota, 243.

Taylor, A.E., Jagger, S., Toplis, P, Wellock, I.J. and Miller, H.M., J. (2013) Are compensatory live weight gains observed in pigs following lysine restriction during the weaner phase? *Livestock Science*, **157**, 200-209.

Tokach, M.D., Goodband, R.D., Nelssen, J.L. and Keesecker, D.R. (1992) Influence of weaning weight and growth during the first week post-weaning on subsequent pig performance. In *Proceedings of the American Association of Swine Practitioners*, University of Minnesota, pp 409.

Toplis, P., Wellock, I.J., Almond, K., Wilcock, P. and Walk, C.L. (2013) Feed intake in young pigs and its importance for the post-antibiotic era. *The Pig Journal*, **69**.

Trckova, M., Faldyna, M., Alexa, P., Sramkova Zajacova, Z., Gopfert, E., Kumprechtova, D., Auclair, E. and D'Inca, R. (2013) The effects of live yeast Saccharomyces cerevisiae on post-weaning diarrhoea, immune response and growth performance in weaned piglets. *Journal of Animal Science*, **92**, 767-774.

Vignola, M. (2009) Sow feed management during lactation. In *Proceedings of the 9th London Swine Conference*, London, Ontario, pp 107-119. Edited by J.M. Murphy.

Whittington, D.L., Patience J.F., Beaulieu, A.D. (2005) Nursery Management and Performance, Prairie Swine Centre Inc. In *Red Deer Swine Technology Workshop*. pp. 44-52.

Walk, C.L., Srinongkote, S. and Wilcock, P. (2012) Influence of a microbial phytase and zinc oxide on young pig growth performance and serum minerals. *Journal of Animal Science*, **91**, 286-291.

Walk. C.L., Santos, T. and Bedford, M.R. (2014) Influence of superdoses of a novel microbial phytase on growth performance, tibia ash, and gizzard phytate and inositol in young broilers. *Poultry Science,* **93**, 1172-1177.

Walk, C.L., Chewning, J. and Wilcock, P. (2014) Influence of the zinc to phytate ratio and superdoses of phytase n piglet growth. *Animal Society of Animal Science - Midwest Meetings*, Des Moines, IA. US, Abstract 159.

Walk, C.L., Wellock, I.J., Toplis, P., Chewning, J. and Wilcock, P. (2014) Influence of increasing pharmacological ZnO dose to 3500 ppm and superdoses of phytase on piglet growth performance and fecal scores from d 0 to d 21 post-weaning. *Animal Society of Animal Science- Midwest Meetings*, Des Moines, IA, US, Abstract 351.

Wellock, I., Toplis, P., Almond, K. and Wilcock, P. (2013) New applications in nursery nutrition and management: Giving piglets the best possible start with practical management tips and nutrition concepts. In *Proceedings of the 13th London Swine Conference*, London, Ontario, pp 155-169, Edited by J.H. Smith.

Wellock, I.J., Wilcock, P., Toplis, P., Chewning, J. and Walk, C.L. (2014) Influence of increasing pharmacological ZnO dose to 2500 ppm and superdoses of phytase on piglet growth performance from d 0 to d 21 post-weaning. *Animal Society of Animal Science - Midwest Meetings*, Des Moines, IA, US, Abstract 318.

Wilcock, P. (2009) Fine tuning nursery management to optimize production costs. (2009) In *Proceedings of the 9th London Swine Conference*, London, Ontario, 21-43. Edited by J.M. Murphy.

Wilcock, P., Bradley, C.L., Chewning, J., and Walk, C.L. (2014) The effect of superdosing phytase on inositol and phytate concentration in the gastrointestinal tract and its effect on pig performance. *Animal Society of Animal Science- Joint Meetings*, Kansas City, MO, US, Abstract 761.

Wolter, B. F. and Ellis, M. (2001) The effect of weaning weight and rate of growth immediately after weaning on subsequent pig growth performance and carcass characteristics. *Canadian Journal of Animal Science*, **81**, 363-369.

Wolter, B. F., Ellis, M., Corrigan, B.P. and DeDecker, J.M. (2002) The effect of birth weight and feeding of supplemental milk replacer to piglets during lactation on pre-weaning and post-weaning growth performance and carcass characteristics. *Journal of Animal Science*, **80**, 301-308.

Zerrahn, J.E. (2008) Optimising sow performance using a probiotic. International Pig Topics, **23**, 13-15.

Zyla, K., Mika., M., Stodolak, B., Wikiera, A., Koreleski, J. and Swaitkiewicz, S. (2004) Towards complete dephosphoylation and total conversion of phytate in poultry feeds. *Poultry Science*, **83**, 41175-1186.

12

Fermented Products and Diets for Pigs

HANNE MARIBO, ANNI ØYAN PEDERSEN AND THOMAS
SØNDERBY BRUUN

Pig Research Centre, DAFC, Axeltorv 3, 1609 Copenhagen V, Denmark

Fermenting diets

Fermenting diets under optimum conditions should increase the content of microorganisms in the diet, particularly the content of lactic acid bacteria. If the fermentation is successful, it may also affect the microbiological balance in the gut and also reduce the level of diarrhoea. However, results have shown that if the total diet is fermented, productivity drops as feed intake is reduced (Pedersen, 2001; Pedersen *et al.*, 2002b; 2002c). Fermenting grain and soya bean meal to which inoculums are added also showed a negative effect on productivity (Pedersen and Lybye, 2012). Therefore, it is not recommended to ferment either diets or soya bean meal, but fermenting the grain (wheat and/or barley) increases feed utilization as digestibility of energy improves (Pedersen *et al.*, 2002a; Pedersen, 2006; Pedersen *et al.*, 2009; Pedersen *et al.*, 2010; Pedersen and Canibe,2011) and digestibility of phosphorus in grain increases during fermentation (Pedersen *et al.*, 2010).

The reason for the reduced feed intake of fermented complete diets is not clear, but the level of biogenic amines and organic acids increases through fermentation and may affect palatability of the feed. The pH value of the diet fed to pigs should never be below 4.5. A pH below this is an indication of excessive fermentation of the diet leading to production of compounds that affect feed intake.

When a complete feed is mixed in a tank, it should be fed to the pigs immediately to avoid loss of synthetic amino acids. However, residuals in the pipes will lead to loss of synthetic amino acids; it is assumed that 8 hours in the pipes will lead to total loss of synthetic lysine (Pedersen and Jensen, 2005). Consequently, Danish farmers are recommended to add more protein and synthetic amino acids to diets if they have residuals in the pipes. Loss of amino acids through fermentation can be avoided by adding formic acid (0.2%) or by using liquid feeding systems without residuals in the pipelines.

Fermenting grain

The optimum process is achieved if the grain is fermented in a separate tank. Grain and heated water (approximately 20°C) are mixed and left for five days before being fed to pigs in order to start the fermentation process. When diets are produced, 50% of the fermented grain is used daily, and new grain and hot water should be added once a day (Figure 1).

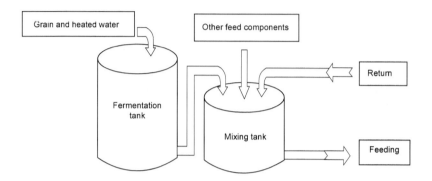

Figure 1. Liquid feeding system with fermentation of grain.

Fermenting grain was investigated in three trials with finishers and one with weaners in different herds. The results demonstrated that feeding weaned pigs fermented grain reduces productivity (Pedersen *et al.*, 2009) probably due to excessive fermentation of the complete diet the pipeline, but improves productivity among finishers (Pedersen *et al.*, 2002a; Pedersen, 2006;Pedersen and Canibe, 2011).

Fermenting grain degrades the fibre that is indigestible for pigs, particularly Non Starch Polysaccharides (NSP), leading to a reduction in dry matter of about 1% and increasing the content of lactic acid. The content of lactic acid in fermented grain is approximately100 mmol per kg liquid feed. Fermenting grain leads to a reduction in the use of grain by 2-3% in the diet as the energy value of fermented grain is higher compared to unfermented grain. Digestibility of phosphorous in grain is also increased by fermentation.

Fermentation of rape seed

The nutritional value does not improve when rapeseed cake is fermented – quite the contrary. Weaner diets (from 9 kg) with fermented rapeseed cake must be approximately 11% cheaper than diets with regular rapeseed cake or soyabean meal. Fermented rape seed cake for weaners showed a reduction in productivity of approximately 7-9% compared to soyabean meal or traditional rapeseed cake. This was attributed to lower feed intake and reduced feed utilization (Table 1). The reduced productivity was attributed to two factors: 1) the producer of the product had set the digestibility of protein too high (9% higher than traditional rape seed cake), and 2) probably a higher content of degradation products of glucosinolates due to either the fermentation process or the drying process after fermentation (Maribo and Sauer, 2012).

The procedure for producing fermented rape seed is:

The mixture:

- 50% rapeseed cake (batch, 5 tons)

- 10% wheat bran

- 40% inoculation material: potato peel, molasses, lactic acid bacteria and water

The fermentation process:

- Mixing cart for cattle feed

- Rammed with wheel loader

- Covered with plastic

- Stored for 7 days

- Drying (Spin Flash)

Table 1. Effect of fermented and regular rapeseed cake on performance of weaner pigs

Diet	Control	Fermented rapeseed cake	Traditional rapeseed cake
No. of pigs	546	559	551
Repetitions	43	44	43
Feed intake, feed units/day	1.04	1.02	1.03
Gain per day, g	531[a]	509[c]	533[a]
Feed utilisation feed units/kg	1.96[a]	2.00[c]	1.94[a]
Index of productivity	100	93	102

a, b Means with different superscripts differ (P<0.05)

Digestibility of fermented rape seed

To confirm these results, a fermented co-product mixture (EP 100) that contained rapeseed meal, wheat bran, soya molasses, and potato peel was tested in a digestibility trial with weaned pigs. The trial comprised seven soyabean and rapeseed protein products and the outcome formed the basis of a revision of table values for raw materials.

Data presented here only include crude protein in dehulled soyabean meal, Scanola rapeseed expeller and EP 100. Fermented co-product mixture (EP 100) had a significantly lower protein digestibility than traditional rapeseed cake and soya protein (Table 2), which explains the reduced productivity value for weaners. However, the production process and composition of the fermented co-product mixture (EP 100i) has been changed, and thus, EP 100i will be included in a new digestibility trial.

Table 2. Protein digestibility of soyabean and rapeseed protein products

Product	Dehulled soyabean meal	Scanola rapeseed cake	Fermented rape seed (EP 100)
Protein digestibility	0.880[a]	0.795[b]	0.706[c]

a-c Means with different superscripts differ (P < 0.05).
1 Data are least square means of 15 observations for all treatments.

With the design of this trial, it was possible to implement standard ileal digestibility (SID) of crude protein and amino acids for soyabean and rapeseed protein products with numerical values in the feed ingredient table. The trial was not designed to analyse productivity and diarrhoea. The trial was conducted at the University of Illinois, using weaned piglets (9.3-19.5 kg) that were surgically equipped with a T-cannula in the end of ileum (Bruun, 2014).

Conclusion

It is recommended to use fermentation of grain for finishers to increase digestibility. Fermenting soya protein or full diets is not recommended either for finishers or weaners as fermentation leads to lower feed intake and feed utilisation. Fermenting rapeseed cake or meal has not been shown to result in protein digestibility that is higher than when using traditional rapeseed cake; productivity was actually lower leading to a reduced value for diets to which fermented rape seed was added.

References

Maribo, H. and Sauer, C. (2012) *Fermenteret raps til smågrise.* Trial report no. 942.
Pedersen, A.Ø. (2001) *Fermenteret vådfoder til smågrise.* Trial report no. 510, Pig Research Centre. www.vsp.lf.dk.
Pedersen, A.Ø. (2006) *Fermented grain for weaners.* Trial report no. 728, Pig Research Centre. www.vsp.lf.dk.
Pedersen, A.Ø. and Canibe, N. (2011) *Fermentering af korn giver en lille stigning i energiværdien.* Trial report no. 895, Pig Research Centre. www.vsp.lf.dk.

Pedersen, A.Ø., Canibe, N., Jespersen, L. and Gori, K. (2011) *Identifikation af mælkesyrebakterier og gær i vådfoder til smågrise.* Trial report no. 919, Pig Research Centre. www.vsp.lf.dk.

Pedersen, A.Ø., Canibe, N. and Lybye, M. (2011) *Ingen effekt af udvalgte podekulturer i vådfoder til smågrise.* Trial report no. 920, Pig Research Centre. www.vsp.lf.dk.

Pedersen, A.Ø., Canibe, N., Poulsen, H.D. and Knudsen, K.E.B. (2009) *Fermenteret korn til FRATS-grise.* Trial report no. 844, Pig Research Centre. www.vsp.lf.dk.

Pedersen, A.Ø. and Jensen, B.B. (2005) *Nedbrydning af syntetiske aminosyrer ved fermentering af vådfoder.* Trial report no. 501, Pig Research Centre. www.vsp.lf.dk.

Pedersen, A.Ø., Jørgensen, H., Knudsen, K.E.B., Canibe, N. and Poulsen, H.D. (2010) *Fermentering af korn øger fordøjeligheden af næringsstoffer.* Trial report no. 873, Pig research Centre. www.vsp.lf.dk

Pedersen, A.Ø. and Lybye, M. (2012) *Fermenteret vådfoder med podekultur øger ikke produktiviteten.* Trial report no. 934, Pig Research Centre. www.vsp.lf.dk.

Pedersen, A.Ø., Maribo, H., Jensen, B.B., Hansen, I.D. and Aaslyng, M.D. (2002a) *Fermenteret korn i vådfoder til tungsvin.* Trial report no. 547, Pig Research Centre. www.vsp.lf.dk.

Pedersen, A.Ø., Maribo, H., Canibe, N., Hansen, I.D. and Aaslyng, M.D. (2002b) *Fermenteret vådfoder til slagtesvin – hjemmeblandet med valle uden myresyre.* Trial report no. 566, Pig Research Centre. www.vsp.lf.dk.

Pedersen, A.Ø., Maribo, H., Canibe, N., Hansen, I.D. and Aaslyng, M.D. (2002c) *Fermenteret vådfoder til slagtesvin – pelleteret foder.* Trial report no. 567, Pig Research Centre. www.vsp.lf.dk.

Sønderby Bruun, T., Vinther, J., Sloth, N.M. and Tybirk, P. (2014) *Digestibility of soy and rape seed products for weaners.* Trial report no. 993. Pig Research Centre. www.vsp.lf.dk.

13

Highlights of the 2012 Swine NRC

BRIAN J. KERR - ON BEHALF OF THE SWINE NRC 2012
COMMITTEE

USDA-ARS-National Laboratory for Agriculture and the Environment, Ames, IA, USA

Introduction

In conjunction with the Animal Nutrition Series developed by the National Research Council of the National Academies, a committee at the end of 2009 was appointed and initiated efforts towards the revision of the 1998 Swine NRC, beginning in January 2010. It had been approximately 14 years prior to the last revision (10th edition, NRC 1998) and even longer since the literature review included in 1998 revision. The committee was comprised of: L. Lee Southern, Chair, Louisiana State University Agricultural Center, Baton Rouge; Olayiwola Adeola, Purdue University, West Lafayette, Indiana; Cornelis F. M. de Lange, University of Guelph. Ontario; Gretchen M. Hill, Michigan State University, East Lansing; Brian Kerr, Agricultural Research Service, U.S. Department of Agriculture, Ames, IA; Merlin D. Lindemann, University of Kentucky, Lexington; Phillip S. Miller, University of Nebraska, Lincoln; Jack Odle, North Carolina State University, Raleigh; Hans H. Stein, University of Illinois, Urbana-Champaign; and Nathalie L. Trottier, Michigan State University, East Lansing.

The committee was charged with a specific statement of task to tackle the process of the revision. The statement highlighted the need to: incorporate information documenting amino acid (AA) needs for modern lean genotypes, identify new knowledge relative to energy utilization especially related to net energy, include description of novel ingredients from the biofuel industry, estimate digestible phosphorus requirements and concentrations in feed ingredients, review the role of feed additives in swine diets, document effects of feed processing on nutrient utilization, identify strategies to increase nutrient retention and thereby reduce nutrient excretion, consider (based on the current status of available information) development of a computer model to estimate nutrient requirements; and expand/refine feed composition tables. In addition, the committee was instructed to highlight future research needs.

The 11th edition of the Nutrient Requirements of Swine, released July 2012 (NRC, 2012), represents a major revision of the previous publication and includes 400 pages, 17 chapters, 5 appendixes, expanded feed composition tables, and a downloadable computer model. The breadth of the publication provides a scientific basis for the resultant requirement estimates, and potential users are encouraged to review the Swine NRC 2012 for this information. For the purposes of the current chapter, only the major points of the revision will be highlighted.

Energy

Chapter 1 outlines energy nutrition of growing and reproducing pigs, and focuses on developing concepts incorporated in the mathematical models described herein and highlighting research investigating energy metabolism in the pig. It should be emphasized here that energy partitioning, as reflected in the requirements developed for all classes of swine, were defined by the models.

Feed energy

It was a priority to develop a feed ingredient database from the scientific literature. Similarly, the establishment of ingredient NE values was viewed as paramount, but because directly determined NE values largely did not exist, an alternate approach was utilized. Initially, the committee pursued the approach to predict ingredient NE values using equations that incorporated digestible energy-yielding components as independent variables. Although these equations were more consistent with animal biology and robust (compared to equations incorporating only component concentrations), the paucity of available literature data (digestible component values) did not support use to predict NE values for ingredients in the database. Therefore, the following equation was used to predict ingredient NE values (all concentrations are expressed as g/kg dry matter (DM); EE, ether extract; CP, crude protein; ADF, acid detergent fibre):

$$NE (kcal/kg) = (0.700 \times DE) + (1.61 \times EE) + (0.48 \times Starch) - (0.91 \times CP) - (0.87 \times ADF)$$

Noblet *et al.*, 1994

Although a majority of ingredients had documented proximate analyses that allowed NE estimation, many ingredients had missing proximate components and thus alternative sources of compositional data were consulted. In the tables of feed ingredient composition (NRC 2012), there is no differentiation of energy for different classes of pigs within ingredient (i.e., for each ingredient one set of energy values is used for starting pigs, growing-finishing pigs, and sows). The amount of published data was considered insufficient to justify differentiation by stage of production.

Components of heat production

Total heat production is partitioned into heat increment, maintenance, heat generated during activity, heat generated to maintain body temperature, and heat arising from waste formation. Clearly, activity and temperature adjustments are typically done by adjusting the maintenance requirement. These adjustments can be significant, but will not be discussed here (see Chapter 1, NRC 2012). Otherwise, if pigs are housed in thermo- neutral conditions with little activity, metabolizable energy (ME) for maintenance can be partitioned accordingly:

ME_m = fasting heat production (FHP) + Heat Increment (maintenance).

As defined in the models, unique estimates for ME_m relative to body weight (BW) are provided for growing-finishing (197 kcal (0.824 MJ)/kg $BW^{0.60}$), gestating (100 kcal (0.418 MJ)/kg $BW^{0.75}$), and lactating sows (110 kcal (0.460 MJ)/kg $BW^{0.75}$).

Physiological states

The essence of describing energy utilization focuses on the partitioning of ME intake (MEI) once ME_m and the associated adjustments are made. For the growing finishing animal MEI is typically predicted using a generalized bridges function (Schinckel et al., 2009):

$MEI = a \times \{1 - \exp [- \exp (b) \times BW^c]\}$.

This equation can be parameterized (a, b, and c values) to predict MEI for different sexes and pigs with differing genetic capacities for growth. The utilization of MEI can be expressed as:

$MEI = ME_m + (1/k_p) PEG + (1/k_f) LEG$,

where, k_p and k_f are the partial efficiencies of ME use for protein (PEG) and lipid energy gain (LEG). Thus, it is critical to accurately define k_p and k_f (model assumes k_p = 0.53 and k_f = 0.75). In the Swine NRC 2012, provisions are also made to consider growing-finishing pigs fed ractopamine and immunizing intact males against GnRH.

The primary determinant of energy use for the gestating sow is litter size and growth (birth weight.) during gestation. Energy can be used directly from MEI (assume k_c = 0.50) or from body lipid mobilization (if MEI < ME_m; k_r = 0.80). Energy deposited supports not only the fetus, but all associated tissues comprising the developing conceptus (e.g., mammary, placenta and fluids, uterus). If MEI > ME_m and ME for conceptus, sow/gilts will deposit fat tissue.

Similarly, for the lactating sow, milk energy output (in addition to ME_m) defines ME requirements. Daily milk energy output is a function of litter size and litter average daily gain (ADG) (Milk energy [GE, kcal/day] = [4.92 × ADG] – [90 × litter size; multiply by 0.004184 for MJ; Noblet and Etienne, 1989]. It is recognized that MEI can be insufficient to meet these needs and body lipid must be mobilized. The efficiency of ME use for milk production was previously estimated to be 0.72 (NRC, 1998). Presently, k_m is set at 0.70 (NRC, 2012). The conversion of body tissue for milk energy (k_{mr}) ranges in the literature from 0.84 to 0.89 and was set at 0.87 in the lactation model. Metabolizable energy intake is predicted using a nonlinear function (Schinckel *et al.*, 2010) and adjusted to reflect differences due to parity.

Effective ME

In concept, current NE systems are more accurate than ME and DE systems in representing the impact of dietary energy source (e.g., starch, fibre, protein, fat) on the efficiency of using dietary energy for supporting animal performance. However, in these NE systems, the purpose for which energy is used by pigs is not considered explicitly. For example, when the NE content in a diet for growing pigs is established, it is assumed that the relative use of energy for protein and lipid gain and for body maintenance functions does not differ between groups of pigs, even when these groups of pigs vary in rate and composition of BW gain. However it is known that the marginal efficiency of using ME for lipid gain is substantially higher than using ME for protein gain and body maintenance functions. In more accurate energy systems, both the dietary energy source and the use of energy by pigs are considered. The latter is accommodated in models that represent the utilization of energy-yielding nutrient in pigs explicitly (Birkett and de Lange, 2001a,b,c; van Milgen *et al.*, 2001). An important limitation of such more mechanistic models is that the (net) energy values of ingredients and nutrients are not constant and are influenced by the animal's performance level, which is difficult to account for in diet formulation.

As a compromise between current NE systems and more mechanistic energy utilization models, the concept of effective ME is adopted in the models that are presented in this publication. In this approach, the effective ME contents of diets are calculated from the diet NE content using fixed conversion efficiencies for either starting pigs (5 to 25 kg BW; 1/0.72), growing-finishing pigs (25 to 135 kg BW; 1/0.75), or sows (1/0.763). These fixed conversion efficiencies are established from calculated NE and ME contents of maize and dehulled solvent-extracted soybean meal-based reference diets that are assumed to be equivalent to diets that have been used for deriving marginal efficiencies of using ME for the various body functions. In the models, effective ME is used to represent partitioning of energy intake between requirements for maintenance, protein, and lipid energy gain, energy gain in products of conception, and milk energy output. When using the concept of effective ME, the effective ME content is higher than the actual ME contents in diets that have low heat increment of feeding (e.g., diets with large amounts of added fat) and lower than the actual ME contents in diets with high heat increment of feeding (e.g., diets that contain high levels of fibrous ingredients). In a similar manner, fixed conversions are used when converting (effective) diet DE content to effective ME content (0.96 for starting pigs, 0.97 for growing-finishing pigs, and 0.974 for sows).

Amino acids

Chapter 2 outlines the protein/AA content of feeds and the description of AA requirements. The utilization of amino acids by growing-finishing and reproducing pigs is defined by the physiological requirement and the efficiency of utilization. Requirements can and are expressed on the basis of dietary concentration, amounts per day, and(or) per unit of metabolic BW ($BW^{0.75}$). The bioavailability of AA from feedstuffs and expressing the potential of AA used for biological functions are typically expressed in terms of ileal digestibility. These indices would include standard ileal digestibility (SID) and apparent ileal digestibility (AID). The estimates of AA requirements are based on needs for maintenance plus productive (tissue) needs. The patterns (ideal profile) of AA are expressed relative to lysine. Optimum ratios are expressed in terms of specific depots/losses and were developed from the literature.

Previously, AA requirements were established based exclusively from empirical values. In the current revision, requirement estimates were critically evaluated from the literature and summarized. Stringent criteria were established in order to consider specific studies (e.g., basal diet definition, multiple levels of the test AA, and identification of appropriate statistical models). These empirical data sets defining AA requirements were used to challenge the model outputs defining AA needs (Figure 1).

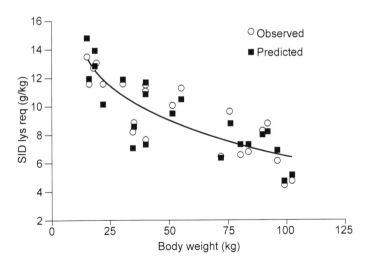

Figure 1. Standardized ileal digestibility lysine requirements observed from 15 studies and predicted with the pig growth model, NRC (2012).

Maintenance

Although the primary factors contributing to amino acid/nitrogen requirements have been defined (see Moughan, 1999; basal endogenous intestine losses, skin and hair AA losses, AA catabolism associated with minimal protein turnover), minimal data exist to quantify these losses. Amino acid requirements for these functions were estimated based on quantity/pattern of AA in the tissue and the appropriate post absorptive utilization.

Growth

Amino acids supplied in excess of maintenance are used for body protein deposition. Therefore, rates of protein deposition (PD), the composition of PD, and the efficiency of SID AA intake for protein deposition must be determined. Critical data sets were used to establish g lysine per 100 g PD (7.1 g lysine/100 g lysine) and AA composition of PD relative to lysine (g AA/100 g lysine).

Gestation

The previous revision (NRC, 1998) only considered maternal and fetal gains during gestation. In addition, AA accretion was based on the pattern established for growing-finishing pigs. In the 2012 NRC, the protein pools were expanded to include; fetal, mammary, placenta, and uterus. Although in many instances the data were limiting or nonexistent, protein accretion versus time (day) were developed.

Lactation

The estimation of milk protein output is driven by litter size and litter growth rate: Milk nitrogen output (g/day) = 0.0257 × mean litter gain (g/day) + 0.42 × litter size. The overall AA needs are balanced between maternal body mobilization and milk protein output.

Minerals

The requirements for the microminerals and macrominerals other than Ca and P will not be discussed. The committee had extensive discussions on Ca and P nutrition and, as a result, a large deviation from the previous NRC (1998) occurred for Ca and P requirement estimates. For growing-finishing pigs, whole-body P needs were predicted from whole-body N content (Figure 2).

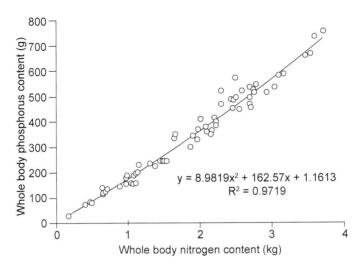

Figure 2. Relationship between whole-body phosphorus and whole-body nitrogen content in growing-finishing pigs, NRC (2012).

Models were then used to establish STTD P and total Ca, with factorial estimates of requirements for STTD P and total Ca are provided in tables for starting, growing-finishing, gestating and lactating pigs. Calcium requirements are based on P deposition and assumed to be a fixed conversion based on physiological state and tissue needs.

A factorial approach similar to that used for growing-finishing pigs was used to estimate STTD P and total Ca requirements for gestating and lactating sows. In general, protein deposition in fetal (including placental fluids), milk, and maternal tissues (including mammary) was the factor driving P content and retention.

Models

A number of the key model elements (growing-finishing, gestation and lactation) have been discussed previously. The three NRC (2012) models to estimate nutrient requirements of growing-finishing pigs, gestating sows and lactating sows are dynamic, mechanistic and deterministic. The models are <u>dynamic</u> because changes in energy utilization and nutrient requirements are represented on a daily basis. This is in contrast to the NRC (1998) sow model in which only mean values across entire gestation or lactation periods were considered. As a result, daily changes in nutrient requirements can be assessed for the development of phase feeding programs for specific groups of pigs, especially growing-finishing pigs and gestating sows.

For estimating nutrient requirements across days or body weight ranges, means of daily requirements are calculated. The models can be considered <u>mechanistic</u> because the underlying biological functions that contribute to nutrient requirements are represented in part, largely in terms of protein and lipid deposition in various pools. These aspects are described in more detail in the next section. The models are <u>deterministic</u> because estimated nutrient requirements represent mean requirements for groups of animals without explicitly representing between-animal variability. However, between-animal variability is considered implicitly in the models by adjusting estimates of post-absorptive efficiencies of nutrient utilization, which is discussed later in detail; these efficiencies are lower for groups of animals than in individual animals (e.g., Pomar *et al.*, 2003). However, differences among groups in between-animal variability are not considered in NRC (2012).

The models are used to represent the partitioning of energy intake - which can be defined on a DE, ME, or NE basis – and to then estimate SID amino acid, STTD phosphorus and total calcium requirements. In the models, estimates of AID AA and ATTD phosphorus requirements are derived from SID AA and STTD phosphorus requirements, respectively. For corn and soybean meal-based diets, estimates of total dietary AA and phosphorus requirements are generated as well. Nutrient requirements of pigs below 20 kg BW and requirements for vitamins and minerals other than phosphorus and calcium have been estimated empirically and are integrated in the models for completeness.

With the NRC (2012) publication, a relatively user-friendly computer program is available that includes the aforementioned models. To run the program, Microsoft Excel™ is required. The computer program also includes the ingredient data base and a simple feed formulation routine, which allows for a direct comparison of calculated diet nutrient contents with model-generated estimates of nutrient requirements. The program also allows direct comparisons between model-generated estimates of animal performance – based on the partitioning of energy intake - and observed performance. Confidence in model-generated estimates of nutrient requirements is generally greater when model-predicted performance is similar to observed performance. To evaluate observed performance of growing-finishing pigs, information about local carcass evaluation schemes may be specified and default values for typical Canadian and USA carcass grading systems are included. The program includes a User Guide and case studies to illustrate the use of these models.

Feed ingredient composition

The feed ingredient data base for the NRC (2012) was completely revised to update contents and availabilities of components in feed ingredients. An exhaustive review of the literature was conducted to arrive at the component/proximate composition of each ingredient with focus on the last 15 years. For apparent and standardized ileal digestibility of amino acids and apparent and standardized total tract digestibility of phosphorus, the time of publication was not considered and an attempt was made to locate every publication that contained these data.

The data base contains 122 feed ingredients, not including fats, mineral sources, amino acids and feed additives, and approximately 130 component or proximate analyses data points. Information on co-products was expanded. For each of the feed ingredients, all information is now presented on an individual page. For all nutrients and proximate components, if the number of observations is included along with a standard deviation (if the number of observations was greater than one), the information is based on the review of the literature. If the number of observations is not presented, then the information was obtained from other summarized sources (NRC, 1998, 2007; Sauvant et al., 2004; CVB, 2008; AminoDat, 2010).

The data on proximate components and carbohydrates are almost exclusively from the review of the literature with the following exceptions. The information for starch and acid detergent fibre either came from the literature review or from other summarized data. Other summarized data were used for these components when necessary because these data were used to calculate net energy. A value for ether extract is presented in this section, and an ether extract value also is presented in the fatty acids section. Although the laboratory methodology was not always clearly described in the published literature, it was assumed that ether extract values came from petroleum ether extraction while and acid ether extract refers to acid hydrolysis methodology. Information about contents of various carbohydrate fractions - starch, lactose, sucrose, various oligosaccharides, crude fibre, neutral detergent fibre, ADF, as well total soluble and insoluble dietary fibre - and fatty acids has also been expanded.

The AA content expressed on a total basis is entirely from the review of the literature or NRC (1998). The apparent digestibility of amino acids is from the review of the literature or other summarized sources. The SID values reflect that amino acids that disappear from the hindgut are not available to the pig and are corrected for the basal ileal endogenous AA losses. A benefit of using standardized ileal digestibility over apparent ileal digestibility is that standardized ileal digestibility values are more likely to be additive among feed ingredients, which is important in diet formulation (Stein et al., 2007).

The total concentration of minerals came from the review of the literature or from NRC (1998). The microminerals are almost exclusively from NRC (1998). The apparent and standardized total tract digestibilites of phosphorus were exclusively from the review of the literature. The use of digestibility measures to estimate bioavailability of phosphorus, rather than bioavailability (NRC, 1998; slope ratio) was considered to be more repeatable and less prone to bias. The use of standardized total tract digestibility values for phosphorus is consistent with the use of standardized ileal digestibility values for amino acids (Stein *et al.*, 2007).

There was almost no new information on the concentration of vitamins in feed ingredients and, thus, these data are almost exclusively from NRC (1998).

The fatty acid data were obtained from Sauvant *et al.* (2004) or from the USDA (2010). The fatty acids are presented as a percentage of ether extract. The ether extract value came from the same source as the fatty acids, and this value was not always identical to the value in the proximate components from the literature review. Iodine value and iodine value product were calculated.

Contents of gross energy, digestible energy, metabolizable energy, and net energy in feed ingredients are presented. Gross energy data are from the literature review or NRC (1998). Digestible energy data are from the literature review, NRC (1998), or Sauvant *et al.*, (2004). Metabolizable and net energy contents were estimated from digestible energy contents, and nutrient and proximate composition (Noblet and van Milgen, 2004). Net energy more accurately reflects the amount of bio-available energy that pigs can derive from feed ingredients, especially from those that contain extreme amounts of fat, fibre and protein.

Research needs

In most energy systems, NE values are predicted from either empirical DE or ME values, from total tract digestibility coefficients (e.g., DM, N, EE, and nitrogen free extract), or from the ingredient's composition. In the current feed database, however, insufficient recent information is available on the content, total tract nutrient digestibility coefficients, or empirical energy values for many ingredients. Consequently, priority needs to be placed on assembling the chemical composition of feedstuffs, determining (bio)availability, which may be estimated from ileal and total tract energy and digestibility, and the development of standardized or reference procedures to estimate their NE content, and subsequent validation with growth performance and body composition indexes. In addition, composition, digestibility, and energy values for various lipid sources, the impact of form (e.g., intracellular versus extracted) on their energy digestibility, and the impact of dietary composition on true lipid digestibility have not been adequately evaluated. Consequently, future research needs to consider all of these factors to advance the understanding of energy digestibility and utilization, and to further the understanding of energy metabolism. In addition, models describing energy utilization to replace existing energy-based (e.g., ME and NE) systems may have the advantage of evaluating evolving and nontraditional feedstuffs (e.g., wet- and dry-milling coproducts) for various body functions more effectively than existing energy prediction equations. This is because of the extreme content (i.e., outside the range of profiles used to parameterize DE/ME/NE prediction regression equations) of these feedstuffs.

Expressions of energy utilization components are considered single unique values; however, variation exists in terms of the specific components (e.g., maintenance, efficiency of energy use for lipid and protein deposition) as applied to populations of pigs that are independent of diet composition and cannot be accounted for relative to current prediction approaches (models). In future research it will be helpful to consider mechanistically defining variation in maintenance energy needs and developing the appropriate predictive equations.

Identifying relationships between energy intake and protein/lipid deposition in growing-finishing pigs, conceptus/maternal tissue accretion/mobilization in gestating sows, and milk production/milk composition/litter performance in lactating sows with various physiological capacities (genetic potentials) need to be explored to improve understanding of energy requirement estimates and modeled responses. Lastly, little data exist describing the effect of immunization of intact males against GnRH or exogenous growth promotants on energy intake and utilization for maintenance and growth.

References

AminoDat 4.0. (2010) Evonik Industries, Hanau, Germany.

Birkett, S., and de Lange, K. (2001a) Limitations of conventional models and a conceptual framework for a nutrient flow representation of energy utilization by animals. *British Journal of Nutrition* 86:647-659.

Birkett, S., and de Lange, K. (2001b) A computational framework for a nutrient flow representation of energy utilization by growing monogastric animals. *British Journal of Nutrition* 86:661-674.

Birkett, S., and de Lange, K. (2001c) Calibration of a nutrient flow model of energy utilization by growing pigs. *British Journal of Nutrition* 86:675-689.

CVB (Dutch PDV [Product Board Animal Feed]). (2008) *CVB Feedstuff Database*. Available online at http://www.pdv.nl/english/Voederwaardering/about_cvb/index.php. Accessed on June 9, 2011.

Moughan, P. J. (1999) Protein metabolism in the growing pig. Pp. 299-331 in *Quantitative Biology of the Pig*, I. Kyriazakis, ed. Wallingford, UK:CABI.

Noblet, J., and Etienne, M. (1989) Estimation of sow milk nutrient output. *Journal of Animal Science* 67:3352-3359.

Noblet, J., Fortune, H., Shi, X. S., and Dubois, S. (1994) Prediction of net energy value of feeds for growing pigs. *Journal of Animal Science* 72:344-354.

Noblet, J, and van Milgen, J. (2004) Energy value of pig feeds: Effect of pig body weight and energy evaluation system. *Journal of Animal Science* 82:E229-E238.

NRC (National Research Council). (1998) *Nutrient Requirements of Swine*. Tenth Revised Edition. National Academic Press, Washington, D.C. 20418 USA.

NRC (National Research Council). (2012) *Nutrient Requirements of Swine*. Eleventh Revised Edition. National Academic Press, Washington, D.C. 20418 USA.

Pomar C, Kyriazakis. I., Emmans, G. C., and Knap, P. W. (2003) Modeling stochasticity: Dealing with populations rather than individual pigs. *Journal of Animal Science.* 81:E178-186E.

Sauvant, D., Perez, J. M., and Tran, G. (2004) Tables of composition and nutritional value of feed materials: Pig, poultry, sheep, goats, rabbits, horses, fish, INRA, Paris, France, ed. Wageningen, the Netherlands: Wageningen Academic Publishers.

Schinckel, A. P., Einstein, M. E., Jungst, S., Booher, C., and Newman, S. (2009) Evaluation of different mixed nonlinear functions to describe the feed intakes of pigs of different sire and dam lines. *Professional Animal Scientist* 25:345-359.

Schinckel, A. P., Schwab, C. R., Duttlinger, V. M., and Einstein, M. E. (2010) Analyses of feed and energy intakes during lactation for three breeds of sows. *Professional Animal Scientist* 26:35-50.

Stein, H. H., Sève, B., Fuller, M. F., Moughan, P. J., and de Lange, C. F. M. (2007) Invited review: Amino acid bioavailability and digestibility in pig feed ingredients: Terminology and application. *Journal of Animal Science* 85:172-180.

U.S. Department of Agriculture, Agricultural Research Service. (2010) USDA National Nutrient Database for Standard Reference, Release 23. Nutrient Data Laboratory Home Page. Available online at: http://www.ars.usda.gov/ba/bhnrc/ndl. Accessed on August 10, 2011.

van Milgen, J., Noblet, J., and Dubois, S. (2001) Energetic efficiency of starch, protein and lipid utilization in growing pigs. *Journal of Nutrition* 131:1309-1318.

14

Feed Processing Technology to Improve Feed Efficiency in Pigs and Poultry

CHARLES STARK, PH.D.

Department of Grain Science and Industry, Department of Animal Sciences and Industry, Kansas State University, USA

Introduction

Producing meat, milk, and eggs to feed 9 billion people by 2050 will be a challenge for the feed and livestock industries worldwide. This challenge will require feed mills to evaluate new technology that will process more by-products from the food and bio-fuels industries into animal feeds. While there have been significant technological changes in feed mills over the last 100 years, the core feed manufacturing processes of grinding, batching/dosing, mixing, and pelleting have withstood the test of time.

The objectives of pig and poultry feed manufacturing are to grind cereal grains to improve digestion, and to combine by-product ingredients from food processors, renders, and bio-fuels industries to create a safe, high quality feed that optimizes animal and bird performance. The adoption of new technology in the feed industry has occurred at a much slower rate as compared to the food industry. The greatest opportunity for improvement may be in the area of data management, specifically the application of statistical process control (SPC) to the feed manufacturing process. Feed mills continue to get larger with more processes being monitored and controlled through the automation system. Koeleman (2014) stated, "More and more things are measured in the feed mill (such as) temperature and moisture content of raw materials before and after they go into the conditioner or extruder. But the challenge is how to deal with the data, otherwise it has no value." The slower rate of adoption may be due in part to the lower profit margins associated with commercial feed sales or the fact, that within an integrated animal production system, the feed mill is simply a cost center charged with delivering nutrients to animals.

Development of new technology or adaption of technology from other industries is often driven by consumer demands and government regulations. Feed mills must often compete for capital expenditures in large corporate environments, which is difficult when the return associated with improved animal performance or increased feed sales is sometimes difficult to measure.

Improvements in the feed manufacturing process have occurred over time as researchers have gained a better understanding of the digestive system of animals and the nutrient requirements of food producing animals. Although advances in technology may occur at a slower rate and take longer to implement, the feed industry must continuously look for new technology that can improve feed quality, feed efficiency of animals, as well as feed mill efficiency. The manager and plant engineer should systematically evaluate each process within their feed mill and look for technology that can be implemented from the time ingredients are purchased to when feed is delivered to the farm. This evaluation must be a coordinated effort between the purchasing agent, nutritionist, and feed mill manager while working with the animal producer to understand their feeding requirements. Whether the feed mill is manufacturing feed to support an integrated production system or selling commercial feed, the objective should be to produce feed that optimizes the production of meat, milk, and eggs.

This chapter will focus on technologies and systems that add value to the feed manufacturing process through improved feed mill operations, animal performance, and feed delivery systems.

Quality control

The foundation of any feed manufacturing facility is the quality assurance (QA) program. Developing a comprehensive QA program is only the first step in the production of a safe, high-quality feed. The production of a quality feed requires the commitment of management, operators, and maintenance personnel. The QA program should contain policies and procedures for purchasing ingredients, receiving ingredients, grinding grains, batching and mixing feed, pelleting, and delivering feed. The most critical procedure is to purchase ingredients from approved suppliers and monitor the quality of the received ingredients. Ingredient specification sheets provide guidance to purchasing agents, suppliers, transporters, and receiving personnel and have always been the cornerstone of producing high quality finished feed, limiting product liability, and lowering the cost of feed (Stark, 2013).

Automation systems

The technology programmed into automation systems continues to develop at a very rapid pace. The new automation systems allow feed manufacturers too closely monitor the feed manufacturing process. In the past, systems would turn on equipment, route ingredients and feed, and maintain basic processing data. However, new systems provide graphics on equipment motor loads, data on operator efficiency, hours of operation for preventive maintenance programs, bearing and rub block temperatures, bar code readers, and remote operations. Automation systems also allow users to input the lot number of ingredients at the time of receipt and then track it through the manufacturing process. The amount of data collected by these systems will continue to grow at a very rapid pace, especially since customers are requesting more documentation on how feed is manufactured as part of the overall global food safety initiative.

Combining automations systems with near infrared (NIR) technology is the next logical step for feed mills. The feed mill manager, nutritionist, and quality assurance personnel now have the ability to monitor nutrient content of ingredients, particle size of ground grains, and nutrient content of finished feed, either with in-plant or in-line NIR. The incorporation of NIR into the QC process will help insure quality parameters are met during receiving, manufacturing, and delivery.

New NIR particle size calibrations are being developed to determine the size of ground cereal grains, which could lead to a system that would alert the operator to change screens in the hammermill or adjust the roll gap setting. Monitoring the moisture content of finished feed in the mixer and then applying water to the feed would standardize the moisture content of feed pre-conditioning, which would provide a consistent mash prior to conditioning and pelleting can also be accomplished with NIR technology. Finally, monitoring the moisture content of the finished feed and making adjustments to the retention time in the cooler or air flow would help control shrink and improve the quality of the finished feed.

Receiving process

The receiving process is the initial step in manufacturing a safe, high quality feed. Feed mills cannot convert low quality ingredients into high quality feed. Feed mills that have the ability to segregate and manage ingredients based on supplier and/or plant location can capture savings through least-cost formulation if they can develop matrix values specific to a supplier or plant location. Simple, inexpensive quality assurance tests at the point of receiving can help segregate ingredients based on moisture, protein, fat, and starch content. Equipment such as the grain moisture analyzer, NIR, or moisture balance can rapidly determine the nutrient content of an ingredient prior to its receipt; typically, these tests take less than ten minutes. In addition to evaluating the nutrient quality of ingredients, mycotoxin testing can be performed on ingredients prior to unloading the truck if the feed mill suspects a problem based on previous shipments. Mycotoxin testing technology has advanced from semi-quantitative to quantitative analysis using single lateral flow test kits, which has significantly reduced the cost of inbound ingredient testing and allowed the manager to reject ingredients that do not meet purchasing guidelines (Stark, 2013).

The use of NIR technology in the feed mill at the production line, rather than in the traditional wet chemistry quality control laboratory, is becoming more prevalent. The ease of sample preparation and operation has helped these systems find their way into feed mills. The advantages of NIR include minimal sample prep, production line or on-line analysis, high precision, low sample cost, and no chemicals or wastes (Eubanks, 2013). NIR in-line technology has the potential to revolutionize ingredient quality control. Unfortunately, most feed mills only obtain a few probed small samples, which are then used to characterize the entire shipment. However, new in-line NIR technology now allows feed mills to measure the moisture, protein, and fat content of ingredients as they pass across in-line probes. The data can then be used to calculate the nutrient average of the shipment and variation within the shipment. In-line monitoring of ingredients during the receiving process also has the potential to route ingredients to designated bins based on the moisture, starch, protein, or fat content of the shipment. This information could also be used in energy calculation formulas to predict the metabolizable or net energy of an ingredient.

Particle size reduction

Particle size reduction of cereal grains is a small fraction of the overall cost of feed manufacturing. The cost of grinding an ingredient is inversely related to particle size; the cost will increase as the target particle size is decreased. The cost of particle size reduction is dependent on the target particle size and the ingredient that is being ground. Particle size reduction can significantly change the digestibility of cereal grains in both pig and poultry (Goodband *et al.* 2002). Particle size reduction of cereal grains has resulted in improved feed conversion in pigs (Wondra *et al.* 1995; Paulk *et al.* 2011; De Jong *et al.* 2012). However, over-processing of cereal grains for broilers has led to poor absorption and gut health issues due to the lack of reverse peristalsis in the bird's GI tract (Chewning *et al.* 2012; Xu, 2013).

The target particle size of cereal grains in pig diets has changed from 600-800 microns to 300-500 microns in the last several years. The benefits of particle size reduction have been well documented over the last 20 years. Wondra *et al.* (1995) reported a linear improvement in feed conversion as the corn fraction of the diet was reduced from 1000 to 400 microns, resulting in an 8% improvement. These improvements have been confirmed in recent studies by conducted by Paulk *et al.* (2011) and De Jong *et al.* (2012) on modern genetics lines. Paulk reported a 4% improvement in feed conversion when the particle size of sorghum was reduced from 724 to 319 microns. De Jong *et al.* (2012) reported a similar 4% improvement in feed conversion in the finishing phase when the particle size of corn was reduced from 650 to 320 microns.

Several studies conducted with broilers have not shown the same positive results to fine grinding the cereal fraction of the diet. Over-processing of the cereal grains in broiler diets appears to have a negative impact on gizzard development, nutrient digestion, and bird performance. Chewning *et al.* (2012) reported a positive advantage of large particles in meal feed, but it tended to diminish when the diet was fed in pelleted form. Svihus *et al.* (2004) and Amerah *et al.* (2007) also reported benefits in bird performance when a wheat-based meal diet contained larger particles. Recent studies have indicated a correlation between the particle size of corn and gizzard development and feed utilization. Xu (2013) reported larger gizzards relative to BW resulted in improved feed utilization, while Ferket (2000) suggested an improvement in gastric intestinal tract health when large particles of corn were included in the diet of broilers. Nir *et al.* (1994) stated that greater coarseness of feed increased relative gizzard weight while Amerah *et al.* (2008) suggested gizzard stimulation was due to the length of time that the coarse particles resided in the gizzard.

There have been significant changes in the design of both roller mills and hammermills, especially in North America where the trend has been towards producing a finely ground cereal grain for inclusion in pig diets. The selection of a grinder should be based on the type of grains used in the formulas, target particle size, final form of the feed (meal versus pellet), and the animals being fed. The operating costs (electricity, labor, and maintenance) and capital investment should also be taken into consideration when selecting the type of grinder to purchase for the feed mill (Heimann, 2014).

The introduction of 3-pair high and 4-pair high roller mills now offers new options for feed mills that have targets of less than 500 microns for the cereal grains portion of the diet. In the past, a well maintained 2-pair high roller mill could achieve the average particle size of 500 micron. However, in addition to the target particle size of less than 500 microns (dgw), customers are now requesting fewer fine particles in the feed. The reduction in the average particle size of the ground grain has led to problems with the finished meal feed not flowing out of bins on the farm. Cleaning corn prior to roller mill processing is also critical at the lower particle size target. Rocks, stalks, and cobs not only result in additional wear on the equipment, but also force the rolls apart when these materials pass through the rolls.

The North American feed industry has moved towards larger capacity hammermills (375 KW) with rotor diameters greater than 135 cm. The focus has been on reducing the particle size of grains to less than 400 microns, improving the effectiveness of air assist systems, and reducing energy and maintenance costs. Pig producers who feed pelleted diets have moved their target particle size from 400-500 microns to 300 microns in an effort to improve feedstuff digestibility. In order to consistently achieve the low particle size while maintaining high throughput, feed manufacturers are using automation systems to monitor feeder rate and electrical energy consumption. Monitoring these two parameters allows managers to create a predictive maintenance program for replacing the screens and hammers based on a breakeven cost of screens and hammers versus energy costs. The incorporation of a variable frequency drives (VFD) on the hammermill main drive motor has also provided greater flexibility in adjusting particle size based on hammer tip speed.

The selection of the correct particle size reduction equipment is only one part of the production of a target particle size. The screens and hammers on the equipment must be kept properly maintained in order to efficient achieve the target particle size. Anderson (2010) estimated that increasing the preventive maintenance cost of a hammermill by 2.5 times would result in a 24% reduction in the total operating costs due to lower energy consumption per ton of ground material. Similarly, maintaining a sharp groove on the rolls in a roller mill and keeping the belts tight will reduce energy costs while maintaining the target particle size. The tendency of management is to focus primarily on maintenance and labor costs by extending the intervals between hammer, screen, and roll replacement. Additionally, if the feed mill management and employees do not understand the negative impact that these decisions have on animal performance (i.e. poor feed conversion), they could potentially increase the cost of raising animals.

Batching and mixing

The combination of a programmable logic computer (PLC) and variable frequency drive (VFD) controllers has increased traceability of ingredients, as well as the accuracy of ingredient additions during the batching process. Automation systems are moving from merely controlling equipment and routing feed to precision feed manufacturing, ingredient lot tracing, using bar code readers during hand additions, and summarizing process data. The new technology offered by many automation companies has helped companies comply with new government regulations and consumer demands. The use of a VFD in new batching systems is becoming a common practice; new feed mill designs are using one VFD to control multiple batching screws over the scale. In addition to improved accuracy of ingredient addition, the number of jogs required to add an ingredient can be reduced with the proper programming of cut-offs and free fall parameters, which reduces the batch cycle time.

Although many systems include statistical process control programs, often managers do not fully utilize these features to reduce batch cycle time and improve ingredient addition accuracy. The incorporation of basic SPC analysis into an automation program can help the manager and quality assurance department reduce shrink and meet nutrient guarantees. Automation systems can be programmed to report the difference between the amount listed on the master formula and the actual amount of ingredients weighed on the scales. In addition to plotting information on process run charts, calculating the mean and variance, automation systems can provide process capability indices. The Cp and Cpk indices on a histogram are important analytical tools when evaluating the batching process. Both the Cp and Cpk capability indices are used to compare the assigned specification limits (USL and LSL) of the process to the variation that exists in the process. The Cp index compares the assigned specification limit to the variation of the process, while the Cpk also takes into account the off-centering of the process during the batching process (Gygi and Williams, 2012).

Automation systems can perform SPC analysis by ingredient and bin each time a batch of feed is manufactured. The data can then be used to make necessary adjustments to cut-off times, free fall, and jog times to improve batching accuracy. The data is also useful to justify the installation of smaller diameter double flight screws or the installation of a VFD on the batching screw conveyor motors above the scale to improve the accuracy of the system. The cost of not adding enough ingredients in an integrated and commercial feed mill will result in poor animal performance and loss of customers, respectively. Whereas the over addition of ingredients results in ingredient shrink.

Thermal processing

Thermal processing traditionally been used with pelleting, expansion, and extrusion. A significant amount of feed fed to animals throughout the world undergoes some type of thermal processing. Pig and poultry research studies clearly indicate that pelleted feed improves animal performance. Animal producers and feed mills must work together to establish a specification for the maximum percent of fines at the feeder, which impacts growth performance and feed conversion. Schell and van Heugten (1998) reported poorer feed conversion in grower pigs as the level of fines in the diets increased from 3% to 40%. Nemechek *et al.* (2012a) reported that feeding pellets versus meal diets improved feed conversion of pigs by 14% in late finishing diets. Additionally, the researchers observed finishing pigs fed screened pellets had the best feed conversion, pigs fed meal had the poorest feed:gain, and pigs fed a mixture of 50% fines and 50% pellets were intermediate. Similarly, Stark (1994) reported that feeding pelleted pig finishing diets, which contained 600g fines/kg, resulted in a feed conversion ratio that was similar to feeding a meal diet, thus negating the benefit of pelleting the feed.

While feed form is important to animal performance, the feed mill manager and animal producers must not overlook the value of feeder management at the farm. Inconsistency in the level of fines delivered to the farm will create additional feeder adjustment as farm personnel attempt to prevent feed wastage. Continually adjusting feeders due to varying levels of fines is often a complaint of customers and animal production specialists. Monitoring the feeders will minimize feed wastage and improve feed efficiency in finishing pigs. Research has shown that monitoring the feeder gap and pan coverage is especially important in heavier pigs (Nemechek *et al.* 2012a). Nemechek *et al.* (2012b) also reported that feeder adjustment had a greater effect on feed conversion in finishing pigs as compared to nursery pigs. Therefore, the consistency of pelleted feed leaving the feed mill is just as important as the actual amount of fines in the feed in order to minimize feed wastage. The installation of an in-line sampler that can systematically obtain samples throughout the loading process will aid the feed mill in determining the percentage of fines for each shipment of feed.

Research studies conducted with broilers have reported improvement in feed conversion when birds were fed pellets versus mash feed (McKinney and Teeter 2004; Lemme *et al.* 2006; and Amerah *et al.* 2007). McKinney and Teeter (2004) suggested there was no advantage to producing more than 40% pellets unless pellet quality was in excess of 60%. Hu *et al.* (2012) reported that birds fed crumbles in any quantity versus mash exhibited a higher feed intake. The higher feed intake resulted in a greater BW when birds were fed in cages; however, most of the positive effect on BW due to feed intake that occurred from feeding high quality crumbles was no longer apparent at 35 d of age after the broilers were moved to the floor pens. These findings were similar to other researchers who reported the addition of fines to broiler diets reduced growth in all diet phases (Nir *et al.*, 1995; Svihus *et al.*, 2004; Corzo *et al.*, 2011). Pacheco *et al.* (2013) reported that as the amount of fines in the feed was increased from 0 to 500 g/kg, there was a decrease in the BW that was not related to feed intake, but associated with a decrease in energy digestibility (0.62 versus 0.60, respectively).

Traditionally, heat treatment has occurred prior to pelleting, but there is new thermal processing and cooling technology that can heat treat feed to be fed as mash diets. However, most feed mills continue to use the pelleting process to reduce pathogens, increase the density of the feed, and reduce segregation of ingredients during transport and feeding. Most pellet mills are equipped with short-term conditioners. The short-term conditioner that steam conditions feed for 20 to 30 seconds is being replaced with conditioners that condition feed for longer than 60 seconds. The change to long term conditioning is being driven by government regulations and consumer demands for greater heat treatment of all feeds. Long term conditioning is being accomplished in a wide variety of ways. The first option is to stack multiple conditioners on top of each other to increase retention time. Typically, this involves two or three conditioners with a retention time of 30 to 45 seconds for each conditioner. Additionally, a VFD is added to the conditioners to maximize the percentage of conditioner fill based on the amps of the main drive motor. Since conditioner fill and retention time are based on production rates, the automation system can be programmed to adjust the conditioner shaft speed based on a feedback loop from the main drive motor. The second option, which is an adaptation of the first option, is to merely increase the size of the conditioner, both in diameter and length, in an effort to increase retention time. Although these two methods can increase the conditioning time from seconds to several minutes, the latest development in conditioning systems incorporate direct steam addition into a pre-conditioner and then utilize indirect heat trace on the conditioner shell.

These new long term conditioning systems are becoming more prevalent as a method to control pathogens in feed in Europe, as well as in North American feed mills that produce feed for broiler breeders. These systems can be used to condition the feed for 5 to 8 minutes at a set temperature, and with proper computer controls, not allow the product to exit the conditioner until it reaches the target temperature. The process can be set up to insure that all of the feed is heat processed to a minimum temperature before entering the pellet mill. In addition to being installed over pellet mills, some companies are using these systems to heat process their meal diets, which are then cooled in a two-stage counter-flow cooler. While heat processing can be used to minimize pathogen levels in feed, there is a growing concern that long term heat processing will reduce amino acid digestibility (Wamsley and Moritz, 2013). Companies who use long-term heat processing should regularly monitor enzyme recovery levels if the enzymes are added prior to the heat processing step.

New technologies in the conditioning process have been driven primarily by feed safety and improved pellet quality concerns. However, there have also been changes in the design of pellet mills, moisture monitoring, roll-speed monitoring and adjustments, and die design. The latest generation of pellet mills have included more sensors and the ability to auto adjust some parameters without stopping the machine (Muller, 2013). The direct drive pellet mill with variable die speed is a recent technology that is being tested in several North American feed mills. In addition to direct drive technology pellet mills, manufacturers are now measuring the speed of each pellet roll to monitor roll slip and make necessary roll gap adjustments. Pellet die manufacturers are also working with new alloy combinations to improve the strength of the die and increase the number of holes and open area in an effort to improve throughput while maintaining pellet quality. Monitoring the moisture content of the feed with in-line NIR technology during the pelleting process has the greatest potential to improve pellet quality, increase throughput, and improve animal performance.

Pellet durability has traditionally been evaluated at the production line with the KSU tumbling box (ASAE S269.5) or the Holmen NHP 100 pellet tester. The new Holmen pellet NHP 200 tester was designed to automatically sieve the sample, determine the weight of the sample, perform the test, and calculate the percentage of durability, thus minimizing the time required to determine durability. The latest development in pellet durability testing is the Holmen NHP 300, a fully automated in-line tester that obtains the sample directly after the pellet mill to determine pellet durability. The Holmen NHP 300 collects, cools, and sieves the sample, performs the tests, calculates the durability, and exports the data to a computer. The operator can then use the results to make the appropriate adjustments in the pelleting process.

New pelleting technology can help improve pellet quality, but the fact still remains that the pellet operators, feed mill manager, nutritionist, and purchasing agent must be in regular communication. Factors such as changes in the inclusion level of ingredients and die thickness ultimately have the greatest impact on pellet quality and pellet mill throughput (Fahrenholz, 2012).

Feed delivery

The final step in the manufacturing process is the delivery of feed. Feed delivery equipment manufacturers continue to reduce the weight of their equipment in an effort to increase the amount of feed delivered to the farms. The reduction in trailer weight is primarily accomplished with aluminum rims, extruded frames, and lighter-weight aluminum panels. Equipment manufacturers have also increased the diameters of the bottom collection screw, lift auger, and boom, which allow the driver to unload the feed in less time. The installation of GPS systems on delivery trucks allows the dispatcher to know the location of the truck and make adjustments in the schedule to optimize the delivery of the feed. While the feed delivery process may not improve the nutritional value of the feed, worn-out equipment will degrade the quality of pelleted feed during the unloading process. The cost per ton of feed delivery often exceeds the cost of feed manufacturing and therefore the efficiency and cost of the delivery system should be regularly monitored. The combination of GPS and high capacity delivery equipment can significantly reduce the cost of feed delivery.

References

ASAE. (2012) *Densified Products for Bulk Handling — Definitions and Method*. ASAE Standard S269.5. American Society of Agricultural and Biological Engineers, St. Joseph, MI, USA.

Amerah, A. M., V. Ravindran, R. G. Lentle, and D. G. Thomas (2007) Influence of feed particle size and feed form on the performance, energy utilization, digestive tract development, and digesta parameters of broiler starters. *Poult. Sci.* **86**, 2615-2623.

Anderson, S. (2010) Optimizing hammermill efficiency. *Feed Mill Managers Seminar.* US Poultry & Egg Association. Nashville, TN, USA.

Chewning, C.G., C.R. Stark, and J. Brake (2012) Effects of particle size and feed form on broiler performance. *J. Appl. Poult. Res.* **21**, 830-837.

Corzo, A., L. Mejia, and R. E. Loar (2011) Effect of pellet quality on various broiler production parameters. *J. Appl. Poult. Res.* **20**, 68-74.

De Jong, J. A., J. M. DeRouchey, M. D. Tokach, R. D. Goodband, S. S. Dritz, J. L. Nelssen, and L. McKinney (2012) Effects of Corn Particle Size, Complete Diet Grinding, and Diet Form on Finishing Pig Growth Performance, Caloric Efficiency, Carcass Characteristics, and Economics. *Swine Day Report 2012*. Kansas State University Agricultural Experiment Station and Cooperative Extension Service. Progress Report 1074. P. 316.

Eubanks, H. (2013) Expanding the uses of rapid assessment technology for feed production. *34th Western Nutrition Conference*. Saskatoon, Canada.

Fahrenholz, A. C. (2012) *Evaluating factors affecting pellet durability and energy consumption in a pilot feed mill and comparing methods for evaluating pellet durability.* PhD Dissertation, Kansas State University, Manhattan, USA.

Ferket, P. (2000) Feeding whole grains to poultry improves gut health. Feedstuffs.**72**, 12-14.

Goodband, R.D., R.D. Tokach, and J.L. Nelssen (2002) The effects of diet particle size on animal performance. *Kansas State University Extension Bulletin*, MF-2050.

Gygi, C. and B. Williams (2012) *Six Sigma for Dummies*. John Wiley and Sons. Hoboken, NJ, USA.

Heimann, M. (2014) Grinding considerations when pelleting livestock feeds. *Feed Pelleting Reference Guide*. Watt Global Media. Section 3, Chapter 10.

Hu, B., C.R. Stark, and J. Brake (2012) Evaluation of crumble and pellet quality on broiler performance and gizzard weight. *J. Anim. Vet. Advances* **11**, 2453-2458.

Koeleman, E. (2014) Is there much left to innovate in feed technology? *All About Feed*. April 11, 2014.

Lemme, A., P.J.A. Wijtten, J. vanWichen, A. Petri, and D.J. Langhout (2006) Responses of male growing broilers to increasing levels of balanced protein offered as coarse mash or pellets of varying quality. *Poult. Sci.* **85**, 721-730.

McKinney, L.J. and R.G. Teeter (2004) Predicting effective caloric value of nonnutritive factors: I. Pellet quality and II. Prediction of consequential formulation dead zones. *Poult. Sci.* **83**, 1165-1174.

Muller, D. (2013) New technology and feed mill design to improve animal performance, feed safety and competitiveness of manufacturing. *34thWestern Nutrition Conference*. Saskatoon, Canada.

Nemechek, J.E., M. D. Tokach, E. Fruge, E. Hansen, S. S. Dritz, R. D. Goodband, J. M. DeRouchey, and J. L. Nelssen (2012a) Effects of diet form and feeder adjustment on growth performance of growing-finishing pigs. *Swine Day Report 2012*. Kansas State University Agricultural Experiment Station and Cooperative Extension Service. Progress Report 1074. P. 290.

Nemechek, J. E., M. D. Tokach, E. Fruge, E. Hansen, S. S. Dritz, R. D. Goodband, J. M. DeRouchey, and J. L. Nelssen (2012b) Effect of diet form and feeder adjustment on growth performance of nursery pigs. *Swine Day Report 2012*. Kansas State University Agricultural Experiment Station and Cooperative Extension Service. Progress Report 1074. P. 1276.

Nir, I., Twina, E. Grossman, and Z. Nitsan (1994) Quantitative effects of pelleting on performance, gastrointestinal tract and behaviour of meat-type chickens. *Br. Poult. Sci.* **35**, 589-602.

Nir, I., R. Hillel, I. Ptichi, and G. Shefet (1995) Effect of particle size on performance. 3. Grinding pelleting interactions. Poult. Sci. **74**, 771–783.

Pacheco, W. J., C. R. Stark, P. R. Ferket, J. Brake, and A. C. Fahrenholz (2013) Effect of particle size and inclusion level of distillers dried grains with solubles (DDGS) and pellet quality on growth performance and gastro-intestinal tract (GIT) development of broilers. *Poult. Sci.* E-Suppl. **1**, 41.

Paulk, C. B., J. D. Hancock, A. C. Fahrenholz, J. M. Wilson1, L. J. McKinney1, and K. C. Benhke (2011) Effects of sorghum particle size on milling characteristics, growth performance, and carcass characteristics in finishing pigs. *Swine Day Report 2011.* Kansas State University Agricultural Experiment Station and Cooperative Extension Service. Progress Report 1056. P. 282.

Schell, T.C. and E. van Heugten (1998) The effect of pellet quality on growth performance of grower pigs. *J. Anim. Sci.* **76**(Suppl. 1), 185.

Stark, C.R. (1994) *Pellet quality I. Pellet quality and its effects on swine performance.* PhD Dissertation, Kansas State University, Manhattan, USA.

Stark, C.R. (2013) Feed processing to increase performance and profit. *34thWestern Nutrition Conference.* Saskatoon, Canada.

Svihus, B., K. H. Klovstad, V. Perez, O. Zimonja, S. Sahlstrom, and R. B. Schuller (2004) Physical and nutritional effects of pelleting of broiler chicken diets made from wheat ground to different coarsenesses by the use of roller mill and hammer mill. *Anim. Feed Sci. Technol.* **117**, 281–293.

Wamsley, K.G.S. and J. S. Moritz (2013) Resolving poor pellet quality and maintaining amino acid digestibility in commercial turkey diet feed manufacture. *J. Appl. Poult. Res.* **22** (3), 439-446.

Wondra, K.J., J.D. Hancock, K.C. Behnke, R.H. Hines, and C.R. Stark (1995) Effect of particle size and pelleting on growth performance, nutrient digestibility, and stomach morphology in finishing pigs. *J. Anim. Sci.* **73**, 757-763.

Xu, Yi (2013) *Interaction of dietary coarse corn with litter conditions on broiler live performance and gastrointestinal tract function.* Ph.D. Dissertation, North Carolina State University, Raleigh, USA.

15

Gilt Management and Nutrition: An Overview

LIA HOVING[1], SIMON TIBBLE[2] AND PATRICIA BECKERS[3]

[1] Species solution manager swine EMEA, Provimi B.V., Cargill; [2] Global Swine Nutrition Manager, Provimi, Cargill; [3] Global Swine Technology leader, Cargill

Introduction

Due to genetic progress sow production has increased dramatically over the past decade. Depending on country, the number of piglets born alive has increased by 1 to 2 piglets per litter resulting in an increase of 2.0 to 4.5 piglets weaned per sow per year (Table 1). Increased production levels put more and more pressure on the sow as a producer of milk and meat. As a result, sow feeding and management practices need to keep evolving constantly, not only to support optimal piglet growth, but also to maximise sow longevity.

Table 1. Increase in number of piglets born alive and weaned per sow per year over the past decade for the United Kingdom, Ireland and The Netherlands. Source: Bpex, Aetagc, Agrovision B.V.

Country	2003 Born alive/litter	2012 Born alive/litter	2003 Weaned/sow/year	2012 Weaned/sow/year
United Kingdom	10.9	11.9	21.5	23.6
Ireland	11.0	12.6	22.8	25.7
The Netherlands	11.6	13.9	23.3	27.9

Besides optimal gestating and lactation feeding strategies, (nutritional) management of the replacement gilt has a large influence on sow productivity and longevity. Since gilts are the future sow herd, optimising gilt rearing, and also management of the young pregnant gilt, are crucial for a long productive life.

This chapter describes management and nutritional factors related to replacement gilt rearing. The authors are aware that most studies are from the 1990s and early 2000s; however, only a limited amount of research has been done with modern genetics. Wherever possible, the literature will be related to practical recommendations while taking into account recent trends in improving sow genetic potential.

Replacement gilt development

Age, body weight and body composition at first insemination are well established factors affecting sow reproductive performance and longevity. However, selection for lean growth and large litter sizes has changed the physiological characteristics of gilts, which might invalidate previous standard practices in the pig industry (Table 2). The modern lean gilt is much leaner and at a lower proportion of her mature body weight at time of insemination compared to her counterpart 20 years ago, which makes her more sensitive to nutritional (mis)management during rearing (Bortolozzo *et al.*, 2009) with the risk of impairing her lifetime performance. The known effects of age, body composition and body weight at first insemination as well as growth rate during rearing, on gilt and sow productivity and longevity will now be discussed.

Table 2. Traditional recommendations for desired gilt body condition at first insemination (in order of importance). Adapted from Close (2003) and Whittemore (1998).

What	Recommendation
Back fat (P2, mm)	18-20
Weight (kg)	130-145
Number of oestrus at first insemination	2nd or 3rd
Daily live weight gain (DLWG, g/day, birth-service)	600-650
Age (days)	210-230

Effect of age at first insemination on reproductive performance and culling

The age of gilts at first oestrus is often used as an indicator of gilt fertility, since gilts that show oestrus at a relatively young age are often the most fertile females in a herd. However, this is only true when good heat detection scheme is in place. In addition, age at first insemination is influenced largely by the number of replacements gilts available and needed. High replacement rates, as can be seen in modern sow herds, often reduce age at first insemination. The effect of age at first insemination on reproductive performance and culling will now be considered.

Importance of early puberty attainment

Puberty attainment is the start of gilt reproductive life and is governed by maturation of the hypothalamic–pituitary–ovarian axis. Once gilts have attained puberty they are physiologically ready to be inseminated. A young age at puberty can therefore be economically interesting since inseminating gilts at a young age lowers costs of the non-productive life. However, it might not always guarantee good reproduction results and a high lifetime production. Even though the modern gilt is able to conceive and produce acceptable first litters at a relatively young age, she may not have enough body reserves to produce optimally and remain in the in the herd for several parities thereafter (Rozeboom *et al.*, 1996).

Optimal age at first insemination

Schukken *et al.* (1994) reported that, based on economic models, the optimal economical age at first conception was between 200 to 220 days. Insemination at an older age increased the number of piglets born alive in the first and second litter but decreased age at culling. Similar results were found by Koketsu *et al.* (1999) who concluded that there was no benefit in delaying insemination beyond 230 days. In contrast, Tummaruk *et al.* (2001) reported a 0.1 piglet increase in first parity litter size with every 10 days increase in age at first insemination. Furthermore, increasing age at first insemination resulted in a decrease in percentage of repeat breeding in gilts and a decreased number of culled sows. Babot *et al.* (2003) divided gilt age at first insemination in 7 age classes of 10 days, varying from <210 days to >270 days. Parity at culling was about 0.5 parity lower for gilts mated at an age of <210 days compared with gilts mated between 221-240 days of age (Figure 1). The total number of piglets born alive during the lifetime of the sow reached its peak (≈ 50 piglets) in gilts with a insemination age of 221-240 days, as did average yearly production (≈ 19.5 piglets).

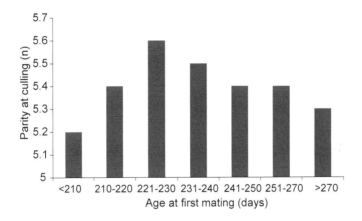

Figure 1. Relation between age at first insemination and parity at culling (adapted from Babot *et al.*, 2003).

From the literature described above, it may be concluded that age at first insemination between 210 and 240 days seems to influence positively reproductive performance in parity 1 and 2. Effects on sow longevity are not as clear. This might be due to the fact that growth, bone and body development during the rearing phase are important factors determining gilt body composition and thereby longevity. Age by itself will therefore not be a good predictor of future reproductive success and increased longevity, and should be combined with gilt body weight, back fat and body protein content as discussed subsequently.

Effects of body composition on reproduction

Besides age, growth rate and body composition influence puberty attainment and sow reproductive efficiency. Growth of gilts comprises accretion of body protein as well as body fat deposition. Growth continues until mature values are achieved; in modern sows around 3rd or 4th parity. In the modern lean gilt, protein accretion and fat deposition are not yet maximised at first service. This results in a gilt with insufficient body reserves at farrowing to meet the (high) energy requirements during first lactation. Studies relating body composition and growth rate during rearing with reproductive performance will now be considered.

Leanness

Selection for maximal leanness, or low back fat, is often thought to be related to reduced fertility, but literature is not consistent. Nelson *et al.* (1990) reported that selection for leanness can be detrimental for reproductive performance. In their study, gilts were selected for high back fat (HB, 19.3 mm, n=13) versus low back fat (LB, 14.5 mm, n=12). More HB gilts showed normal cyclic patterns and gave birth to almost 2 piglets more than LB gilts. In contrast, Patterson *et al.* (2002) found no effect of lean growth on age at puberty. In two experiments, gilts born from either first (Exp 1; n=168) or second parity sows (Exp. 2; n=48) were fed a diet designed to maximize lean growth potential (MLG; n=84 in Exp.1 and n=24 in Exp. 2) or a diet designed to reduce lean growth rate (RLG; n=84 in Exp. 1 and n=24 in Exp.2). The MLG diet increased lean growth from 50 kg to start of stimulation, around day 135 of age (Exp. 1: MLG 424 gr/d vs RLG 347 g/d; Exp. 2: MLG 397 g/d vs RLG 376 g/d), whereas age at puberty was not affected. Negative correlations of around -0.40 were found between age at puberty and growth rate from 50 kg to puberty, indicating that higher growth rate decreased age at puberty. Similar, Kerr *et al.* (1995) and Kerr and Cameron (1996) showed that selection for lean growth did not affect reproductive performance. Selection on low feed conversion ratio or low feed intake, however, did affect farrowing rate, litter size and litter birth weight. In addition, piglet growth rate was negatively influenced by selection for low gilt voluntary food intake or reduced live weight and back fat depth at farrowing. Brisbane *et al.* (1996) studied the effect of different levels of back fat on sow longevity. Gilts and sows were grouped according to back fat (P2) in one of six classes ranging from <10mm to >18 mm, and time of culling was recorded. Compared with the fattest sows, only 67 to

70% of the lean sows survived beyond fourth parity, indicating that lean sows are culled earlier than fat sows.

Fatness

For some time it was thought that gilts had to achieve a certain level of body fatness in order to reach puberty, but literature from the 1990s onwards shows different results. Beltranena *et al.* (1993) studied the effects of energy content of the diet on reproductive performance in gilts. From 75 until 160 days of age, gilts were fed similar diets which differed only in energy content, in order to increase fat reserves. No effect on reproduction was found. From their results, Beltranena *et al.* (1993) concluded that, when protein accretion rate is maximal, differences in body fatness did not influence reproductive development in pre-pubertal gilts. Gaughan *et al.* (1997) studied the effect of body composition at selection on reproductive development. At 145 days of age fifty-four gilts were assigned to one of three groups, based on back fat thickness being either low (L, 10-12 mm); medium (M, 13-15 mm) or fat (F, 16-18 mm). Gilts received the same treatment up to puberty. At puberty no difference was seen in age, weight or back fat depth. L gilts, however, showed a lower number of oestrous cycles and lower number of follicles compared to M and F gilts. Gaughan *et al.* (1997) therefore concluded that selection on leanness might alter the rate of physiological maturation in gilts, but that factors that restrict growth and maturity are probably more important in determining sexual development than leanness. More recently, Williams *et al.* (2005) and Gill (2007) also showed that back fat level at first insemination did not affect number of piglets born during the first 3 parities (Figure 2) or lifetime performance.

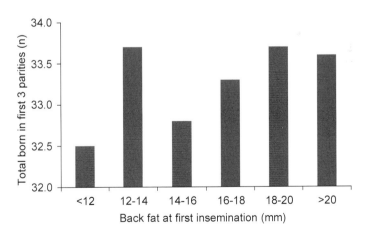

Figure 2. Relation between back fat depth at first insemination and total number of piglets born in the first 3 parities. Adapted from Williams *et al.*, 2005.

Leanness vs. fatness

In order to manipulate lean and fat growth nutritionally, different digestible lysine to net energy ratios are used. In general, feeds with higher lysine to energy ratio stimulate lean growth whilst feeds with lower lysine to energy ratio stimulate fat growth. Cia *et al.* (1998) studied effects of nutritional protein restriction in pre-pubertal animals, in order to obtain larger fat reserves at puberty, on reproductive function. At 118 days of age fifty-four lean genotype crossbred gilts were assigned to three iso-energetic diets with either low (L), medium (M) or high (H) protein concentrations. At 160 days of age the gilts were treated with PG600 and daily examined for oestrous signs. Animals were slaughtered after their second oestrus or at 212 days of age and reproductive tracts were collected. L gilts were lighter, had higher back fat thickness and lower loin muscle depth at slaughter compared to M or L gilts. Ovulation rate at induced oestrus was significantly lower for L (12.5) versus M (17.3) and H gilts (21.5) and a lower proportion of L gilts showed spontaneous oestrus in the subsequent cycle. Cia *et al.* (1998) concluded that larger body fat reserves could be obtained by puberty through protein restriction during rearing, but could negatively influence reproductive performance. In contrast, Stalder *et al.* (2000) did not find any effect of diet composition on reproductive performance. Gilts from 5 different lines, varying in lean growth potential and reproductive capacity, were assigned to one of three diets: 1) High energy and 18% CP; 2) High energy and 16% CP; 3) Normal energy and 23% CP. Diets 1 and 2 were fed from 120 days of age until the gilts achieved a body weight (BW) of 113 kg; Diet 3 was fed from 82 kg until 180 days of age (±100 kg). From 180 days of age onwards, gilts received boar exposure, and gilts in oestrus and older than 210 days of age were artificially inseminated (AI). Developmental diet had no effect on reproductive traits, as measured by number of piglets born total and alive, total and alive litter birth weight, number and weight of piglets weaned.

From the above, one can conclude that age, lean growth or fat growth do not individually have pronounced effects on gilt fertility or lifetime performance, providing they are not too extreme. All these factors should be combined to determine whether a gilt has optimal body composition at first insemination. One could therefore argue that growth (rate), rather than leanness or fatness alone, might influence reproductive performance.

Growth rate and feeding level

Growth and growth rate, measured as weight gain, is a combination of accretion of lean muscle and deposition of fat. Growth (rate) is often steered by feeding level. The effect of growth rate on puberty attainment is established; however the relation with subsequent fertility is not clear.

Simmins (1992) studied the effect of two rearing and three gestation feeding regimes on reproductive performance in sows which were followed for 8 parities. From 10 to 25 weeks of age 156 gilts were fed either 2.25 (L) or 2.7 kg/day (H). Each pregnancy L and H gilts were fed either 1.9 (l), 2.1 (m) or 2.4 (h) kg/day. Even though gestation diet affected weight and back fat at parity eight, no effect of either rearing or gestation treatment on reproduction results was seen. However, the low gestation feeding regime (l) tended to affect longevity, since less l and m sows completed 8 parities compared with h sows (l = 36.5; m = 44.2; h = 52%). Le Cozler *et al.*(1998a; 1999b) studied effects of feeding level, ad libitum vs. 80% of ad libitum, during rearing on performance. They found no effect of feeding level on number of piglets born or piglet and litter weight at birth and weaning. However, age at puberty was 20 to 26 days younger for gilts fed ad libitum compared to gilts fed restrictedly. Ad libitum fed gilts were also heavier and fatter at first service and at farrowing compared with restricted fed gilts. Similarly, Gaughan (2001) studied the effect of three different feeding levels on early reproductive development in gilts and concluded that a restricted feeding level can delay puberty attainment. Gilts were assigned to ad libitum (H) feeding, 75% of ad libitum (M) or 60% of ad libitum (L) from 61 to 176 days of age. Oestrous detection started at 145 days of age with boar exposure commencing at 165 days of age. Average daily gain of gilts was 770 g/d for H, 710 g/d for M and 710 g/d for L. Protein deposition was similar for H, M and L gilts, but H and M gilts had higher lipid deposition compared to L gilts. More H (8 out of 15) than M or L gilts (4 out of 14 for M and 4 out of 15 for L) attained puberty between 145 and 176 days of age. Follicle numbers were similar across treatments; in gilts that attained puberty, however, H gilts had fewer follicles (13.5) compared to M gilts (19.7) and L gilts (21.3). In contrast, Klindt *et al.* (2001a) reported that gilts fed restrictedly from 13 to 25 weeks of age reached puberty fastest. No difference was found in ovulation rate and number of (live) embryos per gilt. At 13 weeks of age, 192 gilts were assigned to one of four pre-pubertal feeding regimes; 87.5%, 75%, 62.5% and 50% of predicted ad libitum energy intake. From approximately 25 weeks of age onwards all gilts were fed ad libitum. Gilts fed 87.5% of ad libitum were heaviest and fattest at first insemination and at slaughter, followed by the 75%, 62.5 and 50% groups. However, average daily gain from 25 weeks of age to pregnancy, when all gilts were fed ad libitum, was higher for the 50% gilts (868 g/d) and 62.5% gilts (746 g/d) compared to the 75% gilts (476 g/d) and 87.5% gilts (405 g/d). Increased growth rate during the last phase probably reduced or alleviated the negative effects on reproduction expected from low feeding levels during the rearing phase. Similar effects were found in an earlier study (Klindt *et al*, 2001b). A large difference between the Gaughan study, which did find effects on reproduction, and both Klindt studies, which did not find effects on reproduction, is that in the Klindt studies gilts were fed ad libitum during the period of puberty attainment. Perhaps the timing and duration of feed restriction determines the effect of feed restriction on reproduction rather than the feed restriction itself.

More recent studies looking at the effect of growth rate on fertility do show a (slight) effect. Kummer *et al.* (2006) combined age and growth rate and reported that gilts with a growth rate of more than 700 g/d and an age of more than 210 days showed higher litter sizes at first parity compared with gilts with a similar age but lower growth rate (<700 g/d) or gilts with a younger age (<210 days) but similar growth rate. Over three parities, however, no effect of age or growth rate on reproductive performance and culling rate was seen. Van Wettere *et al.* (2007) showed that gilts with a growth rate of 800 g/d, from 75 to 175 days of age, had larger follicles at 175 days of age compared with gilts with a growth rate of 500 g/d (Figure 3). Similarly, Chen *et al.* (2011) showed that a higher percentage of gilts on a high feeding level showed follicles of more than 3.5 mm compared with gilts on a lower feeding level. Gilts with larger follicles around insemination will show stronger oestrus and probably also larger litter size. Therefore, one should aim to optimize follicle development around first insemination. Flushing, i.e. feeding insulin stimulating diets, for about 10 day before expected insemination has proven to improve follicle development and can thereby improve litter size.

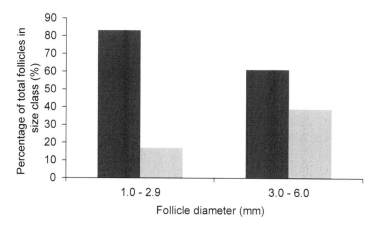

Figure 3. Effect of a low (500 g/d, dark grey bar) or high (8010 g/d, light grey bar) growth rate during rearing on follicle development at 175 days of age (Van Wettere *et al.*, 2007).

Combining age, body composition and growth and its effects on sow production

As discussed above, combining age, body composition and growth rate is necessary to determine whether the optimal gilt rearing has been achieved. Considering lifetime production, Callinor *et al.* (1996) found an increase of 7.2 piglets produced over five parities in gilts mated at a body weight of 130-150 kg and with a P2 of 18-22 mm compared with gilts mated at body weight <120 kg and P2 of 14 to 16 mm. More recently, Stalder *et al.* (2005) reported that sows with back fat >25 mm (at 113 kg) produced more piglets born alive during their lifetime compared to gilts with less back fat, probably because the former remained in the herd for longer. Furthermore, fast growing gilts (>750 g/day) tended to produce more number of piglets born alive during their lifetime versus slow(er) growing gilts, as did gilts with a heavier loin muscle area compared to gilts with a lighter loin muscle area (Stalder *et al.*, 2005). Tummaruk *et al.* (2006) studied the effects of age, bodyweight and back fat on reproductive performance over three parities in 696 gilts. They reported the highest number of total piglets born and born alive in gilts that had a first observed oestrus between 181 and 200 days with 110 to 120 kg bodyweight and 13 to 15 mm back fat. Williams *et al* (2005) showed that gilts with a weight of 135 kg or higher showed the highest number of piglets born in the first 3 parities (Figure 4), whilst back fat was less important (Figure 2). Based on literature reviews, practical experiences and recommendation of breeding companies, the ideal reference points for modern gilts at first insemination have changed slightly, as shown in Table 3.

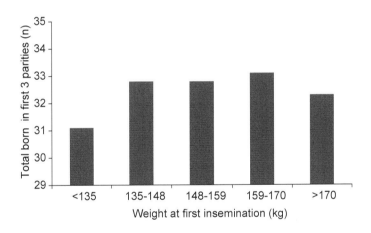

Figure 4. Effect of weight at first insemination on total number of piglet born in first 3 parities. Adapted from Williams *et al.* (2005).

Due to the shift to more lean genetics, weight at first insemination has become more important whilst back fat has become less important. Influencing growth rate in order to have the right weight at the right age is important to prevent animals from becoming too heavy. The use of back fat measurement in gilt rearing, however, should not be discarded. If gilts do not have enough back fat or are too fat, their productivity and lifetime performance will decrease.

The first part of this review has mainly discussed gilt rearing parameters we can affect by either management or feeding. The second part will discuss the role of nutrition in gilt rearing in a more practical way.

Table 3 Current recommendations for gilt condition at first insemination

What	Recommendation
Weight (kg)	135-155
Number of oestrus at first insemination*	2nd
Age (days)	230 (range 210-260)
DLWG (g/d, birth to first insemination)	600-800
Back fat (P2, mm)	15-18

* Not discussed in this chapter, but many studies show that inseminating from the second oestrous cycle onwards gives the most positive results

Role of nutrition in gilt development

Due to genetic selection on finisher characteristics the modern sow has become leaner compared with her counterpart 20 years ago. With the change in leanness it has become fundamental that nutritional programmes during rearing and first parity of the gilt meet the nutrient requirements of the developing gilt. If not met, the risk of sows culled due to reproductive and/or locomotive failures later in life increases. Therefore, nutritional programmes should be developed to fulfil the above criteria, ensuring gilt productivity and longevity beyond 4 parities. The criteria, as mentioned in Table 3, are broad since exact values depend on housing systems as well as breed. As indicated earlier, the modern gilt will continue to grow up to the 3rd or 4rd parity and therefore the nutritional programme must meet requirements for amino acids and energy for body development, calcium and phosphorus for bone development, and vitamins and trace minerals to optimize fertility. Additionally, special attention should be given to fermentable and structural carbohydrates, for their impact on feed intake and behaviour regulation.

Feeding programmes

Historically, replacement gilts have been raised using finisher diets or gestating sow diets, neither of which is formulated to meet the nutrient requirements of the developing gilt.

A finisher diet is designed for fast growing animals with high lean meat deposition, whereas excessive growth rates in gilts may lead to future locomotion problems such as osteochondrosis and leg weakness. Leg problems increase replacement rate within the herd. Furthermore, the vitamins and trace element levels of finisher feed do not support bone development needed for replacement gilts, as will be discussed later.

A gestation diet is designed for a sow that has finished growing and will not meet the amino acid or the mineral requirements of the developing gilt.

Teagasc, Ireland (unpublished data), has recently conducted a trial to evaluate the ideal nutritional programme for gilts. The objective of the trial was to determine the benefit of a specific gilt developer programme, designed to meet the nutritional requirements of the rearing gilt, compared to standard finisher and gestation sow programmes. The trial comprised 100 gilts selected at 55 kg live weight, to determine the effect of three gilt nutritional programmes on gilt performance (Table 4).

Table 4. Feeding programmes tested by Teagasc (Ireland)

Weight Range	Gilt developer*	Finisher diet	Gestating sow
65-100 kg	Developer (restricted**)	Finisher (ad lib)	Finisher (ad lib)
100-130 kg	Developer (restricted**)	Finisher (ad lib)	Gestating (restricted**)
130-140kg***	Developer (ad lib)	Finisher (ad lib)	Gestating (ad lib)

* Gilt developer diets were fortified with organic trace minerals, such as zinc, copper and manganese;
** Restricted = 2.25 kg/day; *** Gilts were slaughtered at 12 weeks of age.

General gilt performance parameters, as well as additional parameters such as locomotory ability, joint abnormalities and bone density at 12 weeks, were recorded. The gilt developer programme significantly reduced lameness (Table 5), as well as claw lesions, claw size and surface lesions on the cartilage of elbow joints.

Table 5. Gilts (%) affected by lameness during the trial period Teagasc (Ireland)

Period	Gilt developer	Finisher diet	Gestating sow
Day 0	0	0	0
Wk 1-4	0	2.2	2.1
Wk 5-8	0	9.1	20.8
Wk 9-12	0	17.7	14.6

Vitamins and minerals

Next to reduced fertility, a major cause of culling in the 1st two parities, representing 25% of total culled sows in a herd, is caused by locomotive problems as defined by lameness, osteochondrosis and claw health. This could be associated with poor mineral supplementation during the rearing period.

The 2012 NRC recommendations show that requirements for calcium (Ca) and phosphorus (P), in order to maximize bone strength and bone ash, desired for replacement gilts, are 0.1 percentage units higher than requirements for optimal gain, wanted for finishers. Besides C and P, Vitamin D and magnesium (Mg) are needed to optimize calcium metabolism and thereby support bone development. Besides the direct effects on culling, lameness has indirect consequences on reproductive performance since it negatively affects production and release of reproductive hormones, apart from the obvious direct causes such as poor lactation, feed intake and physiological changes associated with infection and inflammation.

Although there is limited research on the effect of vitamin and trace mineral supplementation on gilt development, those associated with fertility and immunity are recognized and should be supplemented in a gilt developer programme. Additional Vitamin E and biotin are required to improve hoof development and immune function, while vitamin B6 and Folic Acid are involved in embryo survival and reproductive performance. Supplemented zinc and manganese assists with formation and maintenance of cartilage and bones through synthesis of collagen. In addition, antioxidants can positively affect development of the reproductive system.

Organic trace minerals

The role of organic minerals in a gilt developer programme requires further investigation. The family of organic trace minerals covers a broad range of molecular structures, including chelates, proteinates and amino acids complexes. The differences in mode of action and bioavailability among these chemical forms have still to be studied precisely.

Mycotoxins

Several mycotoxins can influence gilt performance as they can influence sow performance. Zearalone has oestrogenic effects; T2 and DON have potentially negative effects on feed intake; Ochratoxinis are involved with development of gastric ulcers; and Aflatoxin can have an immunosuppressive effect. Considering the above it is important that an effective mycotoxin binder is included in all gilt diets when there is a risk of mycotoxin contamination.

Protein and energy content

Protein (digestible lysine) and net energy values of diets are important for optimal gilt development. Since gilts are growing animals they will need more lysine than gestating sows, but less than fatteners. Energy values should be at such levels that they optimise development without the risk of making the gilt too fat. Finally, manipulating lysine to energy ratio can affect the ratio of lean to fat growth in gilts, which determines body composition at first insemination and thereby reproductive performance of gilts and longevity of sows. In general gilt feed intake is restricted from 15 weeks onwards, but this can be different for every farm and feed. Figure 5 shows an example of general energy and apparent ileal digestible (AID) lysine intake per day for a replacement gilt. Exact values can differ per farm or sow breed. Up to week 10 ($\approx$ 25 kg) replacement gilts can be fed standard starter diets, after which they should switch to specific gilt rearing diets up to the age of 14 weeks. From week 15 ($\approx$ 45 kg) onwards the gilt can switch to a gilt developer diet.

From week 10 to 14 a gilt rearing diet is fed, from week 15 onward a gilt developer diet should be fed.

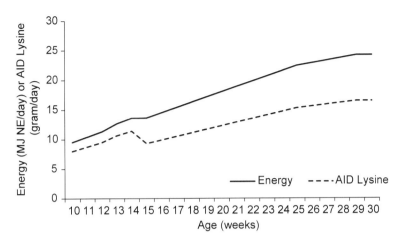

Figure 5. Example of energy and AID lysine intake per day for a gilt from 10 weeks onwards.

Fibre

In addition to energy and protein content, fibre content of diets also affects gilt development. Firstly fibre makes it possible to restrict gilts without the risk on developing stereotypic behaviour. Fermentable fibre in developing diets can increase satiety and therefore reduce the risk on stereotypic behaviour and competition for feed when animals are fed restrictedly. Furthermore, the use of fibre in developer diets also stimulates gut development which is important for transition to gestating diets which often contain substantial amount of fibre. Besides preparing the gut to deal with the higher amounts of fibre in gestating diets, the stomach will also extend and thereby increase feed intake during lactation.

Conclusion

To conclude, gilt rearing should aim to optimise body development, i.e. protein and fat as well as the skeleton and reproductive tract. Considering high productive and lean gilts, weight at first insemination as well as at first farrowing will probably be a better indicator of development than back fat. Weight in combination with back fat is the best indicator of development. Because gilt rearing is the driver of sow heard productivity, a specific gilt rearing and developer diet, containing the right vitamins, minerals, lysine and energy, should be fed. Only then will the gilt have the start she needs for a long and productive life.

References

Babot, D., E. R. Chavez, and J. L. Noguera. 2003. The effect of age at the first mating and herd size on the lifetime productivity of sows. Animal Research 52: 49-64.

Beltranena, E., F. X. Aherne, and G. R. Foxcroft. 1993. Innate variability in sexual development irrespective of body fatness in gilts. J Anim Sci 71: 471-480.

Bortolozzo, F.P., Bernardi, M.L., Kummer, R., Wentz, I., 2009. Growth, body state and breeding performance in gilts and primiparous sows, In: Rodriguez-Martinez, H., Vallet, J.L., Ziecik, A.J. (Eds.), Control of Pig Reproduction VIII, Nottingham University Press, Nottingham, pp. 281-291.

Brisbane, J. R., and J. P. Chesnaus. 1996. Relationships between backfat and sow longevity in canadian yorkshire and landace pigs National Swine Improvement Federation.

Challinor, C. M., A. H. Steward, and S. A. Edwards. 1996. The effect of body condition of gilts at first mating on long-term sow productivity. Animal Science 62: 660.

Cia, M. C., S. A. Edwards, M. Glasgow, S. M., and H. Fraser. 1998. Modification of body composition by altering dietary lysine to energy ratio during rearing and the effects on reproductive performance of gilts. Animal Science 66: 457-463.

Gaughan, J. B. 2001. Effect of restricted feed intake on early reproductive development in large white gilts. Asian-Australian Journal of Animal Science 14: 1534-1541.

Gaughan, J. B., R. D. Cameron, G. M. Dryden, and B. A. Young. 1997. Effect of body composition at selection on reproductive development in large white gilts. J Anim Sci 75: 1764-1772.

Gill, P. 2007. Nutritional management of the gilt for lifetime productivity - Feeding for Fitness or Fatness? London Swine Conference: 83-99

Kerr, J. C., and N. D. Cameron. 1995. Reproductive performance of pigs selected for components of efficient lean growth. Animal Science 60: 281-290.

Kerr, J. C., and N. D. Cameron. 1996. Responses in gilts post-farrowing traits and pre-weaning piglet growth to divergent selection for components of efficient lean growth rate. Animal Science 63: 523-531.

Klindt, J., J. T. Yen, and R. K. Christenson. 2001a. Effect of prepubertal feeding regimen on reproductive development and performance of gilts through the first pregnancy. J Anim Sci 79: 787-795.

Koketsu, Y., H. Takahashi, and K. Akachi. 1999. Longevity, lifetime pig production and productivity, and age at first conception in a cohort of gilts observed over six years on commercial farms. J Vet Med Sci 61: 1001-1005.

Kummer, R., M. L. Bernardi, I. Wentz, and F. P. Bortolozzo. 2006. Reproductive performance of high growth rate gilts inseminated at an early age. Anim Reprod Sci.

Le Cozler, Y., J. Dagorn, J. E. Lindberg, A. Aumaitre, and J. Y. Dourmad. 1998. Effect of age at first farrowing and herd management on long-term productivity of sows. Livestock Production Science 53: 135-142.

Le Cozler, Y. et al. 1999. Effect of feeding level during rearing and mating strategy on performance of swedish yorkshire sows 2. Reproductive performance, food intake, backfat changes and culling rate during first two parities. Animal Science 68: 365-377.

Nelson, A. H., J. W. Mabry, L. L. Benyshek, and M. A. Marks. 1990. Correlated response in reproduction, growth and composition to selection in gilts for extremes in age at puberty and backfat. Livestock Production Science 24: 237-247.

Patterson, J. L., R. O. Ball, H. J. Willis, F. X. Aherne, and G. R. Foxcroft. 2002. The effect of lean growth rate on puberty attainment in gilts. J Anim Sci 80: 1299-1310.

Rozeboom, D. W., J. E. Pettigrew, R. L. Moser, S. G. Cornelius, and S. M. el Kandelgy. 1996. Influence of gilt age and body composition at first breeding on sow reproductive performance and longevity. J Anim Sci 74: 138-150.

Schukken, Y. H. *et al*. 1994. Evaluation of optimal age at first conception in gilts from data collected in commercial swine herds. J Anim Sci 72: 1387-1392.

Simmins, P. H., S. A. Edwards, H. H. Spechter, and J. E. Riley. 1992. Lifetime performance of sows given different rearing and pregnancy feeding regimes. Animal Production 54: 457.

Stalder, K. J., T. E. Long, R. N. Goodwin, R. L. Wyatt, and J. H. Halstead. 2000. Effect of gilt development diet on the reproductive performance of primiparous sows. J Anim Sci 78: 1125-1131.

Stalder, K. J., A. M. Saxton, G. E. Conatser, and T. V. Serenius. 2005. Effect of growth and compositional traits on first parity and lifetime reproductive performance in u.S. Landrace sows. Livestock Production Science 97: 151-159.

Tummaruk, P., N. Lundeheim, S. Einarsson, and A. M. Dalin. 2000. Factors influencing age at first mating in purebred swedish landrace and swedish yorkshire gilts. Anim Reprod Sci 63: 241-253.

Tummaruk, P., N. Lundeheim, S. Einarsson, and A. M. Dalin. 2001. Effect of birth litter size, birth parity number, growth rate, backfat thickness and age at first mating of gilts on their reproductive performance as sows. Anim Reprod Sci 66: 225-237.

Tummaruk, P., W. Tantasuparuk, M. Techakumphu, and A. Kunavongkrit. 2006. Age, body weight and backfat thickness at first observed oestrus in crossbred landracexyorkshire gilts, seasonal variations and their influence on subsequence reproductive performance. Anim Reprod Sci.

Williams, N.H., Patterson, J.L., Foxcroft, G.R., 2005. Non-negotiables in gilt development. Advances in Pork Production 16, 281-289.

Yang, H., P. R. Eastham, P. Phillips, and C. T. Whittemore. 1989. Reproductive performance, body weight and body condition of breeding sows with differing body fatness at parturition, differing nutrition during lactation and differing litter size. Animal Production 48: 181-201.

LIST OF PARTICIPANTS

The forty-sixth University of Nottingham Feed Conference was organised by the following committee:

MR M. HAZZLEDINE (*Premier Nutrition*)
MR R. KIRKLAND *(Volac International)*
MR W. MORRIS (*BOCM PAULS Lt*d)
DR M.A. VARLEY (*Provimi Ltd*)
DR P. WILCOCK (*ABVista USA*)

DR J.M. BRAMELD
PROF P.C. GARNSWORTHY (*Secretary*)
DR T. PARR
PROF A.M. SALTER
DR K.D. SINCLAIR
PROF J. WISEMAN (*Chairman*)

} *University of Nottingham*

The conference was held at the University of Nottingham Sutton Bonington Campus, 24th - 25th June 2014. The following persons registered for the meeting:

Al-Doski, Mr S	University of Nottingham, Sutton Bonington Campus, Loughborough, Leics LE12 5RD, UK
Armstrong, Mr A	Kemin UK Ltd, Tudor house, Hampton Road, Southport, Merseyside PR8 6QD, UK
Bach, Dr A	IRTA, Dept of Ruminant Production, Passeig de Gracia 44 Barcelona 08007, Spain
Bani, Mr P	Catholic University of the Sacred Heart, Largo A. Gemelli, 1, 20123 Milano , Italy
Barile, Ms VL	CRA-PCM, Via Salaria 31, 00015 Monterotondo, Italy
Barringer, Miss C	NWF Agriculture, Wardle, Nantwich, Cheshire CW5 6AQ, UK
Beaumont, Mr D	Lohmann Animal Health, Heinz-Lohmann-Str.4, 27472 Cuxhaven, Germany
Bellet, Miss C	University of Nottingham, Sutton Bonington Campus, Loughborough, Leics LE12 5RD, UK
Birch-Jones, Mr G	Roquette UK Limited, 9-11 Sallow Road, Corby, Northants. NN17 5JX, UK
Blaha, Prof T	University of Veterinary Medicine Hannover, Bueschelewr Str.9, D-49456 Bakum, Germany
Boland, Dr T	Agriculture & Food Science Centre, University College Dublin, Belfield Dublin 4, Ireland
Boyd, Dr P	Premier Nutrition, Brereton Business Park,, The Levels, Rugeley, Staffordshire WS15 1RD, UK
Chagunda, Mr M	SRUC (Dairy Research Centre), Heston House, Dumfries DG1 4TA, UK
Chang, Ms A	University of Nottingham, Sutton Bonington Campus, Loughborough, Leics LE12 5RD, UK
Charman, Mr D	Provimi Limited, Dalton Airfield Industrial Estate, Thirsk, North Yorkshire YO7 3HE, UK

Chiariotti, Ms A	CRA-PCM, Via Salaria 31, 00015 Monterotondo, Italy
Choong, Dr S	University of Nottingham, Sutton Bonington Campus, Loughborough, Leics LE12 5RD, UK
Clark, Mrs G	Roquette UK Limited, 9-11 Sallow Road, Corby, Northants NN17 5JX, UK
Clay, Mr A	Trouw Nutrition, Blenheim House, Blenheim Road, Ashbourne, Derbyshire DE6 1HA, UK
Comyn, Mr S	Techna France Nutrition, Route de St-Etienne-de-Montluc (D101), BP 10 - 44220 COUËRON, France
Down, Mr P	University of Nottingham, Sutton Bonington Campus, Loughborough, Leics LE12 5RD, UK
Dunne, Dr J	Nutriad Ltd, 1 Telford Court, Chester Gates, Chester CH1 6LT, UK
Edwards, Miss J	University of Nottingham, Sutton Bonington Campus, Loughborough, Leics LE12 5RD, UK
Fiandanese, Ms N	Parco Tecnologico Padano, Via Einstein, Lodi, Italy
Fitches, E	Food & Environment Research Agency (Fera), Sand Hutton, York YO41 1LZ, UK
Gabler, Dr N	Iowa State University, 201 Kildee, Ames IA 50011, USA
Garnsworthy, Prof P C	University of Nottingham, Sutton Bonington Campus, Loughborough, Leics LE12 5RD, UK
Goatman, Mr T	DairyCo, AHDB, Stoneleigh Park, Kenilworth, Warwickshire CV8 2TL, UK
Goodman, Miss J	University of Nottingham, Sutton Bonington Campus, Loughborough, Leics LE12 5RD, UK
Gregson, Dr E	University of Nottingham, Sutton Bonington Campus, Loughborough, Leics LE12 5RD, UK
Hawkey, Miss K	University of Nottingham, Sutton Bonington Campus, Loughborough, Leics LE12 5RD, UK
Hawkey, Mr R	Mole Valley Farmers, Moorland House, Station Road, South Molton, Devon EX36 3BH, UK
Hazzledine, Mr M	Premier Nutrition, Brereton Business Park, The Levels, Rugeley, Staffordshire WS15 1RD, UK
Henderson, Mr A	University of Nottingham, Sutton Bonington Campus, Loughborough, Leics LE12 5RD, UK
Homer, Dr E	University of Nottingham, Sutton Bonington Campus, Loughborough, Leics LE12 5RD, UK
Hoving, Dr L	Provimi B.V., Veerlaan 17-23, 3072 Rotterdam, The Netherlands
Huhtanen, Prof P	Swedish University of Agricultural Sciences, Umeå, Sweden
Jacklin, Mr D	RNC, UK
Jagger, Mr S	AB Agri, 64 Innovation Way, Peterborough PE2 6FL, UK

Jones, Miss S	AB Vista Feed Ingredients, 3 Woodstock Court, Marlborough Bus. Park,, Marlborough, Wiltshire SN8 4AN, UK
Kadar, Dr G	Helvecia Protein Trade Kft, Szeghalom, Tildy Zoltán u. 5, 5520, Hungary
Kaprzak, Dr M	University of Nottingham, Sutton Bonington Campus, Loughborough, Leics LE12 5RD, UK
Kerr, Prof B	USDA-ARS-National Laboratory for Agriculture & Env, 2110 University Boulevard, 2165 NSRIC, Ames IA 50011, USA
Kirkland, Dr R	Volac International, 50 Fishers Lane, Orwell, Royston, Hertfordshire SG8 5QX, UK
Kiss, Dr T	University of Pecs, Hungary
Lawson, Dr D	Premier Nutrition, Brereton Business Park, The Levels, Rugeley, Staffs WF15 1RD, UK
Lawson, Mrs K	University of Nottingham, Sutton Bonington Campus, Loughborough, Leics LE12 5RD, UK
Lim, Mrs P	University of Nottingham, Sutton Bonington Campus, Loughborough, Leics LE12 5RD, UK
Lund, Miss E	University of Nottingham, Sutton Bonington Campus, Loughborough, Leics LE12 5RD, UK
Maribo, Dr H	Danish Agricultural & Food Council, Pig Research Centre, L & F, Axelborg, Axeltorv 3 1609 Copenhagen V, Denmark
Marlow, Mr A	Kite Consulting, Dunston Business Village, Dunston, Staffordshire ST18 9AB,
Marr, Miss D	University of Nottingham, Sutton Bonington Campus, Loughborough, Leics LE12 5RD, UK
Masey O'Neill, Dr H	Aunir (AB Agri), 3 Woodstock Court, Blenheim Road, Marlborough Business Park, Marlborough SN8 4AN, UK
May, Miss K	University of Nottingham, Sutton Bonington Campus, Loughborough, Leics LE12 5RD, UK
McDermott, Miss K	University of Leeds, Woodhouse Lane, Leeds LS2 9JT, UK
Menn, Dr F	Lohmann Animal Health GmbH, Heinz-Lohmann-Str.4, 27472 Cuxhaven, Germany
Mohammed, Mrs A	University of Nottingham, Sutton Bonington Campus, Loughborough, Leics LE12 5RD, UK
Mohammed, Mr R	University of Nottingham, Sutton Bonington Campus, Loughborough, Leics LE12 5RD, UK
Mohammed, Mr Z	University of Nottingham, Sutton Bonington Campus, Loughborough, Leics LE12 5RD, UK
Mostyn, Dr A	University of Nottingham, Sutton Bonington Campus, Loughborough, Leics LE12 5RD, UK
Nakagawa, Mr K	Ajinomoto Co. Inc., 15-1 Kyobashi 1-chome, Chuo-ku Tokyo (104-8315), Japan
Newbold, Prof J	IBERS Aberystwyth University, Penglais Campus, Aberystwyth SY23 3DA, UK

Newsome, Mr R	University of Nottingham, Sutton Bonington Campus, Loughborough, Leics LE12 5RD, UK
Nichols, Dr S	Frank Wright Ltd, Blenheim House, Blenheim Road, Ashbourne, Derbyshire DE6 1HA, UK
Noordhuizen, Prof J	Charles Sturt University, Wagga Wagga, NSW 2678, Australia
Northover, Mrs S	University of Nottingham, Sutton Bonington Campus, Loughborough, Leics LE12 5RD, UK
Parr, Dr T	University of Nottingham, Sutton Bonington Campus, Loughborough, Leics LE12 5RD, UK
Partridge, Mr G	Danisco (UK) Ltd, P O Box 777, Marlborough, Wiltshire SN8 1XN, UK
Pomar, Dr C	Agriculture and Agri-Food Canada, 2000 College Street, Sherbrooke Quebec J1M 0C8, Canada
Poole, Dr M	Campden BRI, Station Road, Chipping Campden GL55 6LD, UK
Potterton, Dr S	University of Nottingham, Sutton Bonington Campus, Loughborough, Leics LE12 5RD, UK
Randall, Miss L	University of Nottingham, Sutton Bonington Campus, Loughborough, Leics LE12 5RD, UK
Reynolds, Prof C	University of Reading, School of Agriculture, Policy & Development, Whiteknights, PO Box 237, Reading RG6 6AR, UK
Robinson, Mr M	Sciantec Analytical Services Ltd, Bishopdyke Road, Selby, North Yorkshire YO8 3SD, UK
Rose, Mr D	Carrs Billington Agriculture (Sales) Ltd, Montgomery Way, Rosehill Industrial Estate, Carlisle CA1 2UY, UK
Routledge, Mr I	Carrs Billington Agriculture (Sales) Ltd, Montgomery Way, Rosehill Industrial Estate, Carlisle CA1 2UY, UK
Sakowski, Mr T	Institute of Genetics and Animal Breeding, Poland
Salter, Prof A	University of Nottingham, Sutton Bonington Campus, Loughborough, Leics LE12 5RD, UK
Salter, Mr M	AB Agri Ltd, 3 Blenheim Road, Marlborough, Wiltshire SN8 4AN, UK
Saunders, Mr N	University of Nottingham, Sutton Bonington Campus, Loughborough, Leics LE12 5RD, UK
Schimmel, Mr D	De Heus Animal Nutrition, Rubensstraat 175, Ede 6717 VE, The Netherlands
Sherwin, Miss VE	Univesity of Nottingham, Sutton Bonington Campus, Loughborough, Leics LE12 5RD, UK
Sinclair, Prof K	University of Nottingham, Sutton Bonington Campus, Loughborough, Leics LE12 5RD, UK
Slinger, Miss K	University of Nottingham, Sutton Bonington Campus, Loughborough, Leics LE12 5RD, UK

Stark, Dr C	Kansas State University, Dept of Grain Science & Industry, 201 Shellenberger Hall, Manhattan KS 66506-2201, USA
Taweel, Dr H	Schothorst Feed Research, PO Box 533, 8200 AM Lelystad, Netherlands
Tennant, Miss L	University of Nottingham, Sutton Bonington Campus, Loughborough, Leics LE12 5RD, UK
Tiberghien, Dr D	EFFAB, PO Box 76, NL-6700 AB Wageningen, The Netherlands
van Vuuren, Dr A	Wageningen UR Livestock Research, PO Box 65, 8200 AB Lelystad , The Netherlands
Vickers, Dr M	EBLEX, AHDB, National Agricultrual Centre, Kenilworth, Warwickshire CV8 2TL, UK
Walker, Dr N	AB Vista, 3 Blenheim Road, Marlborough, Wiltshire SN8 4AN, UK
Wallace, Mr J	University of Aberdeen, King's College, Aberdeen AB24 3FX, Scotland
Ware, Mr J	Roquette UK Limited, 9-11 Sallow Road, Corby, Northants NN17 5JX, UK
Webb, Prof R	University of Nottingham, Sutton Bonington Campus, Loughborough, Leics LE12 5RD, UK
Wellock, Dr I	Primary Diets, Melmerby Industrial Estate, Melmerby, Ripon, North Yorkshire HG4 5HP, UK
White, Dr G	University of Nottingham, Sutton Bonington Campus, Loughborough, Leics LE12 5RD, UK
Wilcock, Dr P	AB Vista, 3 Woodstock Court, Blenheim Road, Marlborough Business Park, Marlborough SN8 4AN, UK
Wilcox, Miss R	University of Nottingham, Sutton Bonington Campus, Loughborough, Leics LE12 5RD, UK
Wiseman, Prof J	University of Nottingham, Sutton Bonington Campus, Loughborough LE12 5RD, UK
Yossifov, Mr M	Institute of Animal Science, Kostinbrod at Bulgarian Agricultural Academy, 2232 Kostinbrod, Bulgaria
Zeebaree, Mr B	University of Nottingham, Sutton Bonington Campus, Loughborough, Leics LE12 5RD, UK

INDEX